the
TICK SLAYER

Battling Lyme Disease and Winning

Perry Louis Fields

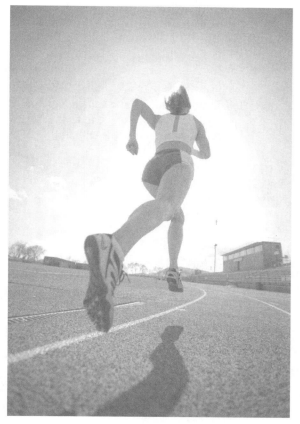

the
TICK SLAYER

Battling Lyme Disease and Winning

Editor: Bree Ervin
Cover Photo, Inside Photos and Design: Joel Strayer
Interior Layout: Andrea Costantine
Inside Illustrations: Perry Louis Fields

ISBN: 978-0-98298-607-3
Library of Congress Number: 2011929584

Category: Health & Fitness/Diseases/Immune System

This book is available at quantity discounts for bulk purchases.
For more information
visit: www.TheTickSlayer.com/bulk

Dedication

This is for everyone everywhere who is tired of being sick. It's for those who are diligently looking for answers and beating their own path to what they want in life. It's for the people who never say NEVER, who search relentlessly for answers.

To the people who choose the harder right, those who don't cast stones so quickly, and those who continue to love despite the challenges.

I've met people who I can honestly say I wouldn't be here without their help, it's these people who gave me something concrete to stand on during my darkest hours. Thank you for believing in me, even when I felt like a failure. Thank you for reinforcing my belief in the cure and in having a full recovery.

For all those who are still searching, **expect nothing less than the best.** This is for you.

CONTENTS

CONTENTS CONTINUED

Contents Continued

I Want to Be the Fastest
Runner in the World!

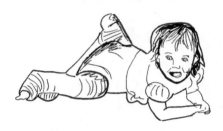

"If you would attain greatness, think no little thoughts."
– Author Unknown

I'm no stranger to obstacles. I spent the first years of my life learning how to walk with one leg 2 inches shorter than the other. How or why I ended up a runner is beyond explanation. It must have been a subconscious desire because ever since I can remember, I've wanted to run...even when I couldn't walk.

At the age when most toddlers learn how to walk, my mother noticed that I kept falling over. I spent over a year in a half-body cast to get my hip back into place, after being diagnosed with hip dysplasia. After the cast came the braces. Not quite the Forrest Gump style of leg braces, but still quite cumbersome. A series of straps and a harness kept me from straightening my legs. Everyone in my family still talks about it.

On a recent trip to my grandparent's house, both of them mentioned how vividly they remember the Christmas I began walking again. They told me how at their house that Christmas, I walked around the entire day, going up to each of my family members and telling them "see I can walk." I had just turned three.

All I remember of the ordeal was the frustration of growing up watching other kids play. My sister, Arden, two years my senior, pulled me to her play spots in a Radio Flyer® red wagon where I would quietly watch, unable to participate. Despite the frustration and having all of my not-so-cute baby pictures dominated by my cast and straps, the treatment worked. My hip dysplasia was fixed and I was able to walk – and run!

I got tough at an early age and nothing got me down for long. With this attitude even the biggest battle of my life, Lyme disease, was just something else for me to conquer, even when it seemed impossible at first.

Lyme disease is now thought to be the fastest growing infectious disease in the world. There are believed to be at least 200,000 new cases each year in the U.S. and some experts think that as many as one in every 15 Americans is currently infected (20 million persons)[1]. Lyme disease is a stealth bacteria spread from the bite of a tick. It is now thought that mosquitoes, fleas, spiders and even human to human contact can pass the bacteria. The Lyme bacteria can sometimes be quickly destroyed when the diagnosis occurs within weeks

1. Dr. James Howenstine, "Curing Lyme Disease With Samento,". http://www.samento. com.ec/sciencelib/4lyme/curinglymewsam.html (accessed September 14, 2011).

and treatment is given, but the problem is that most people never remember being bitten or even know how they got it. Years later, debilitating and life threatening symptoms can surface. Getting a diagnosis is just the first part of the battle, but even with the diagnosis, many people don't get better, and some even die from the disease. Patients who die usually succumb to many health problems, which the disease seems to exacerbate. Lyme can cause extreme inflammation in the body, including in the organs, like the heart, which can lead to an abnormal heart beat and possible heart failure. A late stage diagnosis can cause significant damage, which some believe is irreversible.

A few months ago, I was sent a clip of a documentary about Lyme disease called *Under My Skin* (*www.undermyskin. com*). Watching it made me incredibly emotional. It was hard to watch these people, including other professional athletes and people from all over the country, who were all disabled by a tick tell their stories! Their lives were drastically changed for the worse; some had no hope, others just wanted to end it all, and some were just trying to find reasons to keep going. It was then that I realized what I had done, curing myself of Lyme, was miraculous by many people's standards. I felt compelled to write this story to help others who are crippled by Lyme and other autoimmune diseases find some answers and be inspired by the possibilities.

I had vomited when I had nothing more to vomit, cried when I had no more tears, hoped when there was no hope in sight, fought back when I had no more fight in me, was stretched to the outer limits and had the endurance test of a lifetime. This is the story about what I went through to turn the tide against Lyme disease and to go back to racing in the sport I love, track and field.

Even though I'm cracking the code of chronic (late-stage) Lyme disease in this book, the principles in this story can be applied to anyone with a "mysterious" disease (usually autoimmune related) that the medical world doesn't know how to treat successfully. Because I believe all autoimmune diseases occur in people who have many of the same underlying health issues, a lot of these hidden issues must be examined and corrected to restore one's health. The fundamental issues that need to be addressed are ones that develop from what seems like normal living. The excessive amounts of pollution that our bodies have to deal with on a daily basis, to the nutritionally devoid foods we consume daily, and the stress that most people have in their lives.

What Is Lyme Disease?
An Exploding Epidemic

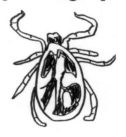

"The only good is knowledge and the only evil is ignorance."
– Socrates

Lyme disease (LD for short) is an infectious disease. Pathogens like viruses (such as HIV), bacteria (Lyme disease), fungi, protozoa and other larger parasites are lumped together under this term. Infectious diseases are often incredibly hard to get rid of. Other infectious diseases are hepatitis, influenza, leprosy, rabies, syphilis, typhoid fever, and giardiasis.

Lyme disease is transmitted by ticks, which prey on infected deer. They have carried the bacteria from the New England states to just about every other corner of the world. Lyme can also be transmitted by fleas, mites and mosquitoes and is now thought to be able to be transmitted from one person to another, either sexually (congenial transfer) or through the placenta to an unborn baby (if the mother is carrying the bacteria). Miscarriages, still births, birth defects and premature births have all been linked to Lyme disease. The Lyme bacteria may also elude detection by blood processing techniques and can be spread through blood transfusions.

There are other ways to get the bacteria beyond what is typically thought. (Which is hiking in the woods, being an avid hunter or outdoor enthusiast and living in areas commonly associated with Lyme disease.) It's important to know that anyone living where there are deer is susceptible to Lyme. Once thought of as a disease you could only get in the New England states, it is now showing up in all 50 states and even worldwide.

The scientific name for Lyme bacteria is Borrelia burgdorferi (or Bb for short). It is spiral shaped (similar to the spirochete that causes Syphilis) and is often accompanied by the bacteria Babesia (a microti parasite) and Ehrlichia bacteria. Many micro organisms can be considered parasitic in that they need a host to survive, but the term parasite usually refers to larger organisms. Bacteria are parasitic in nature, so they are sometimes referred to as parasites. Babesia is a sporozoan (which is also considered a parasite, reproduces via "spores" and is frequently transmitted by bloodsucking insects) and Ehrlichia is a gram-negative rickettsia bacteria carried by many ticks, fleas, and lice, and causes diseases in humans such as typhus, rickettsialpox, Boutonneuse fever, African tick bite fever, and Rocky Mountain spotted fever. One more bacteria, called Bartonella, is also often an accompanying co-infection (this causes "Cat Scratch Fever").

The life cycle of many of these bacteria and the extent

of the damage they cause is unknown. With millions of ticks, other insects, animals and people who can spread the infection, it's safe to say you can pretty much get it anywhere, although it might be highly unlikely at the North Pole!

Lyme disease is the fastest growing infectious disease in the world as of 2009. A Lyme advocate and insurance researcher told me that the Center for Disease Control (CDC) reports about 10% of the actual cases. It's well known among the Lyme community how large the actual number of cases really is. Disease reporting likely underestimates the actual number of cases for a given time period because reporting national notifiable diseases to the CDC is voluntary. Additionally, the completeness of reporting likely varies by disease. This is influenced by many factors such as the diagnostic facilities available, the control measures in effect, public awareness of a specific disease, and the interests, resources, and priorities of state and local officials responsible for disease control and public health surveillance (CDC, 2010).

Many Lyme disease victims who see doctors and are misdiagnosed are told by their doctors they can't get Lyme disease in their state. Tests for positives are poor, and the standards are so conservative that sometimes medical history and symptoms are the only ways to truly get a confirmation of the disease. The last problem is that most people who have it don't even know. Most people never remember being bitten by a tick, (or they got it another way). Ticks are tiny and secret fluids that desensitize the skin to their bite. They need just a small amount of blood, and they drop off when they are done feeding, usually undetected by their victims.

Latent or Chronic cases of these diseases occur when

the bacteria lies dormant or perhaps the immune system has it under control until it comes out with a vengeance. What I have learned is that it rears its head when the host has a weakened immune system, whether from stress, a physical trauma, or just an unhealthy lifestyle. When this happens, all hell breaks loose inside the person carrying the bacteria and they can become deathly ill.

To make matters worse there is conflicting information about the disease and medical groups are pitted against each other. The Infectious Disease Society of America (IDSA) maintains that Lyme is hard to catch, easy to treat and that a normal round of antibiotic therapy is the correct treatment[1]. Dr. Andrea Gaito, M.D., F.A.C.R., former President, International Lyme and Associated Diseases Society (ILADS) contends that ILADS physicians find that 10 days of therapy is not sufficient in preventing the development of systemic manifestations of Lyme disease[2]. One of their physician members contends that "persistent symptoms have been noted in 25%-80% of patients with Lyme disease after 2-4 weeks of antibiotic therapy[3]." This means that many people who find themselves ill with Lyme disease will have a chronic case of the disease, just like me.

There are over 350 conditions that Lyme can be mistaken for or that are connected to Lyme disease such as: Alzheimer's Disease, ALS (Amyotrophic Lateral Sclerosis or

1. The Infectious Diseases Society of America (IDSA) "IDSA: Ten Facts about Lyme Disease," http://www.idsociety.org/Lyme_Facts/ (accessed September 14, 2011).
2. Dr. Andrea Gaito, "Lyme Study in Annals of Internal Medicine Flawed," http://www.ilads.org/about_ILADS/position_papers1.html (accessed September 14, 2011).
3. Raphael B. Stricker, "Counterpoint: Long-Term Antibiotic Therapy Improves Persistent Symptoms Associated with Lyme Disease," Antibiotic Therapy and Lyme Disease CID 2007:45 (15 June) 149.

Lou Gehrig's Disease), Bell's Palsy, CFS (Chronic Fatigue Syndrome), Fibromyalgia, IBS (Irritable Bowel Syndrome), Lupus, MS (Multiple Sclerosis), Parkinson's Disease, Rheumatoid Arthritis, Syphilis, Allergies, Arrhythmia, ADD, ADHD, Autoimmune Disorders, Cognitive Dysfunction, Depression, Migraines, Meningitis, Parkinson's Disease, Dementia and Sleeping Disorders[4]. Know anyone who has any of these? Lyme can induce and mimic symptoms of these and other diseases. Borrelia burgdorferi is believed to be a direct influence on the creation of other diseases such as the development of autism[5]. New York pathologist, Dr. Alan MacDonald, provided evidence of the Borrelia spirochete in extractions of fresh autopsy Alzheimer's disease brain specimens[6].

That's why I believe that in order to recover from many of these diseases you should take the same approach as if you had Lyme disease. A lot of fancy names are given when the body just finally hits failure and is unable to defend itself from assaults (whether chemical, like pollution, or pathogens of various natures).

---

4. Martha Grout, MD. Arizona Center for Advanced Medicine, http://arizonaadvanced-medicine.com/articles/lyme_disease.html (accessed October 3, 2011).

5. Bransfield RC., Wulfman JS, Harvey WT, Usman AI, "The association between tick-borne infections, Lyme borreliosis and autism spectrum disorders." Med Hypotheses. 2008 ;70(5):967-74. Epub 2007 Nov 5.

6. Alan B. MacDonald, "Plaques of Alzheimer's disease originate from cysts of Borrelia burgdorferi, the Lyme disease spirochete," Med Hypotheses, May 2006, Volume 67, Issue 3, Pages 592-600. Alan B. MacDonald, "Alzheimer's neuroborreliosis with trans-synaptic spread of infection and neurofibrillary tangles derived from intraneuronal spirochetes," Med Hypotheses, 2006 Oct 19.Visit www.molecularalzheimer.org for information on Dr. MacDonald's studies.

The Tick Slayer is Born

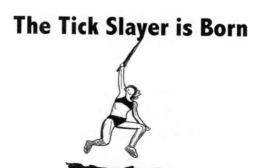

"Nearly every man who develops an idea works it up to the point where it looks impossible, and then he gets discouraged. That's not the place to become discouraged."
– Thomas Edison

At the beginning of this medical journey, I had one big decision to make. I was really ill for only a few months but had gone downhill so fast. I was in terrible pain and I couldn't take care of myself. Getting out of bed was a chore. Staying positive about the situation was tough as my head was constantly combating negative mental chatter about my situation. It wasn't living, it was dying.

I felt like I had two choices. One was to commit suicide and the other was to recover 100% so that I was not limited in any way from doing any sport or activity to the level I desired. From an athlete's perspective, it was all or nothing for me. I couldn't see life without the full use of my body. If I was going to find a way to cure myself, I was going to have to spend an enormous amount of time finding it and I had to have faith that there really was a cure! It's hard to believe that one would think of suicide, but it's hard to describe the loss of desire to live when day to day living becomes excruciatingly painful. Chronic suicide risk is particularly associated with an inability to appreciate the pleasures of life (anhedonia). Suicidal tendencies occur in a high percentage of Lyme disease patients who have brain disorders[1]. (Lyme patients for whom the disease takes on neurological symptoms as well as the physical ones.)

It wasn't like me to give up on anything, so I took the harder right instead of the easier wrong. I was going to cure myself completely.

The greater the highs you go for, the greater the lows you experience and being an athlete has allowed me to experience both often and to be acquainted with the constant extremes. This was just another low. You could say it was a HUGE low. I had to accept that this low was only temporary and it was to be a part of my journey in life; a difficult truth to swallow.

Once I decided I would recover fully, nobody could tell me otherwise and now I can finally say with conviction today, "Yes, I do believe Lyme disease and other autoimmune diseases are completely 100% curable." Those words alone should provide a huge relief to many millions of people who find themselves in this situation. It's the initial weapon you need to begin recovery with. It's the idea that you CAN recover completely.

I've always been an optimistic person but knowing I had

---

1. Robert C. Bransfield, MD, "Lyme, Depression, and Suicide," accessed October 15th, 2011, http://www.mentalhealthandillness.com/Articles/LymeDepressionAndSuicide.htm (accessed October 15, 2011)

such a terrible disease challenged my usual outlook on life. Looking back I believe the darkness I fell into was related to one of the bacterial infections associated with Lyme disease, called Bartonella.

Bartonella is a common co-infection of Lyme disease. This bacterium is associated with rage, depression and mental illness. Bartonella can pass through the blood brain barrier (a cellular structure that restricts the passage of different chemicals and bacteria while allowing important substances for metabolic function to pass through) and disturb the brain's capacity to control automatic actions (like breathing and heart rate), get messages from your senses (like hearing, seeing and tasting), collect and sort information (like remembering an important event or being able to think clearly, which is often a complaint of Lyme patients).

I knew I had the Bartonella bacteria due to my symptoms. The testing (done by serology or PCR) is a very insensitive test. Symptomatic indicators of this bacterium involve the central nervous system being skewed (agitation, anxiety, insomnia, confusion). I also had many red rashes that looked like streaks and had extremely enlarged lymph nodes in the throat and armpits, which are often indicators of this type of bacteria. People who are chronically ill become seriously depressed, but Bartonella can put someone in a mental prison. It takes an emotional toll when you can't take care of yourself and being ill can also keep your body from functioning correctly so having physiological problems due to the loss of internal stability (the breakdown of the body) is common.

Once I made my decision to recover, I had to get my faith back. To do that, I had to control all the uncharacteristic self-defeating babble going on in my head. Athletes are known for pumping themselves up through thick and thin to prepare themselves for workouts and competitions. I had to find that positivity again. I had to start talking to myself just to combat the constant negative feelings that assaulted me daily.

Although I wasn't anywhere close to being able to train again, I knew that blocking the negative mental chatter and creating positive affirmations would be the starting point for my success. I didn't want to bullshit myself, so I really put belief into these affirmations. I told myself that each day was a new day to make more progress and I started writing down what I called my "health calendar" where I would write exactly what I did that day to help me move toward recovery. I would write on the calendar, weeks and even months ahead that I would be having great days. I visualized myself having these days and pictured what a great day for me would really encompass. When I started having days where I felt like I had an inkling of progress, it made me believe even more. The biggest overall affirmation I kept making was that I was going back to track and field, and that I would run better than ever before. I didn't know when, but I knew I was going back, because that would mean that I was cured.

The worst days for me involved just lying on my back for hours at a time, staring at the ceiling. I used this time to visualize myself racing again. I would have vivid dreams of racing with such ease that my talent was finally in full fruition and none of my competitors could touch me. I was telling my body that this was what it was going to be doing again and there was no negotiation. I was creating my destiny.

For a period of time I had terrible nightmares, which I believe were my body and mind's way of overcoming the emotional side of being ill. These nightmares would wake me abruptly; I'd be sweating and unable to control my body temperature. Every night I woke up in hell. To keep from becoming emotionally disturbed about the dreams I was having, I wrote them down and, by doing so, I let them go. My nightmares would put any horror movie to shame. Sometimes I would wake up in pools of sweat thinking that my skin was crawling. I fought armies of ticks in my dreams. They crawled into my bed from between the floorboards and descended from my ceiling onto my bed. Anytime I got depressed about the nightmares I would replace those thoughts with something positive. I started becoming The Tick Slayer in my dreams. The Tick Slayer was a cunning intellectual; she took no prisoners, and was completely fearless of the unknown. She was a true warrior, reminiscent of Boudicca, an Irish female warrior who led uprisings against the Romans in 60 A.D. She wouldn't have been scared of some tick bite and neither was I.

Believing in something positive can assist you in healing. My grandfather, Dr. William Perry (a retired physician), is 99 years old, and he's had everything from a quadruple bypass to cancer to hepatitis C. Just recently, he had an enormous melanoma tumor on his head removed, and if you ask him how he is doing, he'll tell you smiling, "I've never been better."

My recovery wasn't a miracle. It was work that anyone can do if the desire is strong enough. There are so many aspects of the human body that science can't even explain. It's as wondrous as the universe and just as complex. The hope lies in the possibilities, because they are practically endless.

Disaster Strikes Early On

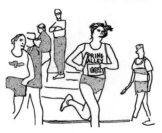

"Acceptance of what has happened is the first step to overcoming the consequences of any misfortune."
– William James

In my senior year in high school, I was hit by a school bus whose driver ran a stop sign. I was in a Volkswagen Jetta®, and a big yellow bus appeared out of nowhere. My friend, a French exchange student, yelled right before the accident happened. I briefly saw the grill of the bus out of the corner of my eye, but it was too late to get out of the way. The woman driving the bus was taking a bunch of elementary kids to the skating rink. I was driving back to school from lunch. The bus driver sat there, frozen, as if her mind had stopped working, and didn't even acknowledge her screaming kids, nor us (good thing we weren't dying). I even made the evening news.

I didn't lose any limbs, because I had that precious second

to react, so I saved my legs from being crushed. The bus hit my side of the car and crushed the back like a can, sending us into a violent spin, ultimately putting us in a ditch. The worst part is that I still vividly remember the shock of the impact. For a few minutes I was completely deaf and blind. I got lucky and was discharged from the hospital with only a few bruised ribs. My friend was completely unharmed. But, the stress of the impact and the whiplash caused severe problems for me.

That was the last time I was truly healthy. Something was triggered that day: Lyme disease, but I was unable to put this together until a decade later. I didn't think about getting tested for a tick bite at age 18 (no one really knew about it). So I carried on. I had severe Chronic fatigue syndrome that started my last year in high school. It was a crap diagnosis. Obviously, fatigue is caused by something, but that is just one of the unfortunate general diagnoses given these days by doctors, afraid to get more hands on. The answers, in my opinion, are always there!

By graduation, I already had appointments to West Point, The Naval Academy and acceptances to every school I wanted to attend. All that hard work my last two years of high school paid off. I was offered approximately $850,000 dollars in scholarship money. I felt relieved that my parents didn't have to pay for my college. I think I was the only person in my school to graduate with every advanced placement honor ribbon there was.

I had been pretty happy-go-lucky until the car accident. I had no beef with anyone. I went to school. I ran. I won.

The only person who became a problem was my high school track coach (who I believe exacerbated my health issues my senior year, especially after the car accident). Like all high school and even college sports programs, you get sucked into winning it all for the team. The team is more important than the individual, which is tough for those kids who are in Olympic sports, where it's really about the individual. It's why I like individual sports and why after excelling in sports growing up, I decided to focus all my efforts in becoming the best in an Olympic sport. If I won, it was because I made it happen. As an athlete, you can't get more satisfaction than that.

Unfortunately, most sports, if not all, require the individual to be part of a team. The end result for someone serious about their athletics is usually extreme malcontent and, if the coach is one of those types who want to win it all, at all cost, then the individual will find themselves used up until there is not much left. Emotionally drained, physically drained and harboring lots of ill sentiment.

In high school I ran multiple events at every meet so I could carry the team to more state titles because at this point the coach hadn't lost a state team title in a decade and the pressure was on me to win it all for her. I was stretched so thin that at every race I was going just to win (not to set records or challenge myself to new personal records). It was misery and this was the first time, and not the last time, that a coach would make track a miserable experience. Winning was easy, putting up with jerk coaches was beyond difficult.

Running in South Carolina was not a joy either. Not a race would go by that I wouldn't hear someone yell, "Don't let that white girl beat you!" This is what it was like. I was a quiet kid, but athletics changed that. I learned to be aggressive and outgoing just to cope with the social and racial pressures.

I ended my high school career on a sour note, emotionally drained from dealing with my coach. I ran poorly after the car accident because I continued to train, thinking that if I didn't run I wouldn't be able to go to college. I ran in pain and was trying to do physical therapy and chiropractic care to correct the whiplash issue.

I know that the day of the car accident was the trigger for my Lyme disease even though I don't know exactly when I was bitten as a child. I was a healthy child up until that point.

Off to College with Brewing Health Issues

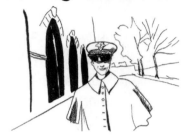

*"Courage is always greatest when blended with meekness;
intellectual ability is most admired when it sparkles in the
setting of modest self-distrust; and never does the human
soul appear so strong as when it foregoes revenge
and dares to forgive any injury."*
– Author Unknown

I was successful in college despite undiagnosed food allergies, a run-in with Epstein-Barr virus, Chronic fatigue syndrome, and the on-going recovery from the car accident. I was always cowgirling up. I just wanted to run!

I ended up deciding on West Point. It was too good of an offer to refuse and I adored Coach Quiller, the head track and field coach. But West Point was a disaster for my health. I had to leave for summer training before school started, and I was still trying to recover FAST from the car accident. Because I continued to run, I actually did more harm than good.

I had developed terrible ear pain due to undiagnosed food allergies. I was eating gluten and oranges almost every day and I was allergic to them. I still had pain due to the car accident, but I wasn't complaining about any of it. I was too busy being a cadet.

The army medical system goes like this: sucking chest wound, we can help! Broken leg, we can help! Foot shot off, we can help! But if you have any strange symptoms, you're popping pills to hopefully make it all go away.

My health issues never went away at West Point. I spent most days walking around in "soft shoe profile," meaning that instead of wearing the West Point issued black leather shoes and boots; I wore running shoes with my uniform. I wasn't the only one with shin splits and shin fractures. Even though lots of other cadets were wearing these, it was seen as a sign of weakness.

I realized that it was time for me to leave West Point early on. I couldn't train with the track team (although I was clearly one of the best recruits they ever had and Lord knows all I wanted to do was run fast). But I was tired of being sick. I couldn't do the thing I wanted most in the world - and that was to run in college and be wildly successful. That's all I really wanted, and I was willing to sacrifice West Point for it. It was the hardest decision I've made so far in my life. I have no regrets; I'm just sorry it didn't work out.

After West Point I wanted to quit school all together. After all I had always hated school, but I ended up going back. My parents were forceful in saying that it was an experience everyone should have. (I beg to differ now that I'm 30 but how could I argue at 19 years of age?)

I transferred to Appalachian State and was only there for a year because the track coach who recruited me left about 11 months later. I was stressed from the news and the thought of changing schools once again. One day after returning from the weight room back to my dorm, I didn't feel so good. The next day, I went to the health clinic and found out I had Epstein-Barr virus (EBV), often referred to as mononucleosis – mono for short) which I believe I picked up in the weight room. Known as the college kissing virus, everyone kept asking me whom I had kissed to get it, but I had never been the promiscuous type and didn't get it from kissing anyone.

The EBV never fully went away (and once I was bitten by the last tick that did me in a few years later, it was reactivated), and the food allergies that were still undiagnosed at this time were still not permitting me to regain my health fully.

In class I had a hard time paying attention, especially after lunch or breakfast (these are the times most people typically eat gluten in foods like bread, cereals, muffins, etc.) Gluten is the sticky stuff that binds flour when you add water. I was lucky to be smart because how I made the grades I did is beyond me. I just remember not being able to pay attention and feeling extremely lethargic during certain classes.

All I knew at this time is that I had Epstein-Barr virus and was diagnosed with Chronic fatigue. I was never an unhealthy child, but I think having a poor diet in my teenage years, undiagnosed gluten intolerance, the stress of athletics at an early age, and the physical stress of the car accident was enough to keep my immune system down so much that I could barely defend myself from any type of pathogen I encountered or any pathogen I had already come into contact with. I had extreme immune deficiency and I was still trying to run in college! I just couldn't let it go. That was the problem, I couldn't quit running because I had already "quit" West Point so that I could run! What a dilemma. I just kept going because I didn't know what else to do.

I left Appalachian State for Clemson University where I ultimately had to settle. I went there because I heard this famous coach, who had coached the world's best middle distance runners (including gold medalists) had just started coaching there and thought, "Is this a dream?" But once I got to Clemson, he was let go after 6 months. Committee members were strong on the opinion of having a woman coach the women[1]. An all star team was recruited and we all found ourselves at a college without the coaches we originally came for and were all pretty steamed. *Ah, CRAP, here we go again...the college coach shuffle!*

In a sport like track and field, where development over the years is key to having a career in the sport after college, a decision like this did nothing for the athletes at Clemson. All it did was fill the needs of a bunch of committee members who felt for some reason they knew what was best for us athletes. Bureaucracy at it's very finest. It happens all the time, in all the universities across the country and can ruin athletes.

I got lucky however with the young "stand in" coach, under the newly hired head coach. Track was REALLY good for about 6 months (I made it all the way to the big show, the NCAA meet, with one of the top mile times in the nation) until the end of the season when I found myself with a very serious case of anemia.

I had been asking our team doctor about making sure my

---

1. Pete Iacobelli, "Take Two For Clemson Hire's White." Herald-Journal, Spartanburg, South Carolina. July 29th, 1999, http://news.google.com/newspapers?nid=1876&dat=1 9990727&id=_T0fAAAAIBAJ&sjid=0M8EAAAAIBAJ&pg=5388,8691510 (accessed October 25, 2011).

iron levels were right and I constantly got the same thing, "here's some Vioxx®." For people who don't know, Vioxx is a pain killer. Looking back, I realize someone should have been checking my iron levels routinely. Not taking care of your athletes is neglect, plain and simple. We should have all had routine blood work and at some university programs they do just that. Athletes should have their blood levels checked regularly as sweating causes the body to lose all kinds of minerals and vitamins.

Once I crashed and really forced someone to check my blood levels, my iron was fatally low and would take a long time to rebuild. Once your storage of iron is depleted it can take months to restore. So I had about 4 months of bliss when I was really shining and felt like I had my game back. After I crashed, it was over. I had no idea the trouble was just beginning.

Looking back, I have to laugh at how sick I really was, not just from anemia but all of the undiagnosed issues like gluten intolerance. I still can't believe I ran as fast as I did in college. I must have been possessed.

In college I thought about being a doctor just like my grandfather and great-grandfather. A love of medicine runs in the family. Never once did a doctor ever tell me that my problems might be from something I was eating! I had to go to a kinesiologist to find out about this possibility and get my gluten intolerance diagnosed. Because of that, I decided not be a doctor. I didn't want to simply write prescriptions all day. I didn't want to be a slave to insurance companies and pharmaceutical reps and I didn't want my peers to look down on me if I found an incredible new way to treat someone.

After changing my diet, my life changed for the better in a dramatic way! All those years of eating gluten and then struggling to have an athletic career despite it, could have been avoided to a large degree. I was even a "space cadet", largely because of my health problems, in my classes and somehow still managed to pull off good grades. Had I not had these problems, I would have probably been the most annoying "A" student of all time (you know the ones that sit in the front row, raising their hand like, "Oh, oh, oh, I know this one").

All those years of eating oranges and grapefruits were the cause of my continuous ear infections. My Chronic fatigue was mostly due to a food allergy (and of course major stress) and anemia is actually quite common in athletes and also very common in women in general. Just having the right balance of iron in your body will do wonders! Your iron storage (Ferritin) should always be tested along with your hemoglobin.

But my tragic college career had really broken my spirit and the worst was still getting ready to happen. Believe it or not, the new assistant coach decided to leave after just one season of coaching. He got us all in shape and took Clemson to a third place team title in 2001 at NCAAs. After he left, our new head coach called me to her office to tell me she thought my talent was a fluke and was thinking about giving my scholarship to a sprinter.

I had to tell her why I deserved the scholarship because apparently being the 2nd fastest miler in Clemson history and the only Clemson middle distance runner to go to NCAA since the 80's wasn't enough. This was the beginning of the end for me as a college athlete and I knew it just from our conversation. What I realized, which was news to me, was that my head coach didn't care about me and didn't believe in me. Her conversation with me took me back to some of my encounters in high school regarding the same poppycock, but this wasn't from some delinquent bystanders in the stadium, it was from my head coach, someone who was supposed to care about me and support me.

I should have just quit track at that very moment, but I didn't want to lose my scholarship. I was trapped. I had nobody who cared about my success and you cannot compete successfully when your own coaches have never coached your event (ever). It was a lost cause and unfortunately I just didn't have the wisdom needed to quit. I was young, brash and bent on proving her wrong, despite my growing medical issues that remained unresolved.

The best part of college track, is that it came to an end. I felt like I was finally free. Once I left college I was ready to rock and roll. I finally had control over my career and my life.

The good news is that my quick achievements in college proved to me that I really was a great athlete. This made me realize I should seek the coach I had originally gone to Clemson for, as he offered to me get ready for the 2004 Olympics under his direction. I went with him to train with his Brazilians and Africans. It was a very good environment for me to be in, especially after the chaos and heartbreak of college athletics. Everyone was nice, cared about each other's success, and provided outstanding training partners.

Pulling the Bloodsucker
Off the Back of My Head

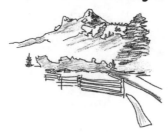

"Fortune brings in some boats that are not steered."
– William Shakespeare

In the summer of 2003 after I graduated, my family went to the North Carolina Highland Games at Grandfather Mountain in the Blue Ridge Mountains. I ran the Celtic mile (tartan optional) and walked around meeting other Scotch-Irish locals and distant "cousins" from overseas. After my race I sat in a shaded forest listening to bands play. I must have sat there with hundreds, if not thousands, of other people that day. It was a pleasant day. The irony of this day bringing about my downfall is not lost on me.

Two days later, I began picking at what I thought was a scab at the nape of my neck at the start of my hairline. Standing in front of the bathroom mirror, I can remember picking to see what it was. Once I got it lose, I looked at it...

HOLY SHIT! It was a tick! I thought I was going to pass out. The tiny reddish brown tick was squirming, so I quickly flushed it down the toilet.

I showed the bite to my mom. This is where I went wrong, telling her, "Well, if I go to the doctor, they won't really know what they are looking at. I don't feel bad at all. I've been bitten by everything at this point and if I get on antibiotics I will have to stop training for the 2004 Olympics."

A week went by and I felt like I might be training too hard. I felt achy. My boobs were killing me, but they always hurt during PMS, and I thought that it must just be that time of the month again. The lymph nodes in my armpits also hurt and I felt like I had a small cold…and then Badda Bing! It was gone completely. I kept training because I had the Olympics on my mind. I thought there was nothing to worry about and I kept going.

Train Away!
2004 Olympics are Coming!

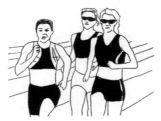

"We risk going too far to discover just how far we can go."
– Jim Rohn[1]

I got ready to leave for Cochabamba, Bolivia, to train at altitude with my new coach, Fun stuff, my bags were packed – I was ready for anything! Other than packs of wild dogs chasing you on runs (which is good for training purposes), the drug trade, and getting depressed from seeing all of the homeless children, it was a fairly good place to train, with a good climate for such a high attitude (about 8,500 feet).

While training in Bolivia and then back in Tucson, Arizona, I noticed a lack of ability to recover. Obviously, this

---

1. Quote from Jim Rohn, America's Foremost Business Philosopher, reprinted with per- mission from Jim Rohn International ©2011. As a world-renowned author and success expert, Jim Rohn touched millions of lives during his 46-year career as a motivational speaker and messenger of positive life change. For more information on Jim and his popular personal achievement resources or to subscribe to the weekly Jim Rohn Newsletter, visit www.JimRohn.com.

was a sign that I was either doing too much or had something wrong. Healthy people can recover quickly from exercise. At this time, I thought I was just training too hard, because I was finally in a program and training consistently. Even being sick with Lyme, I still flourished to a degree, simply because I was with good people, doing what I loved.

At the Olympics Trials, I was quite fit and was the "new girl" for the most part in my event. The only thing I was really uncomfortable with was the fact that I was racing against veterans (ladies who had raced every major international competition the last 8 years), but on the other hand I was thinking "bring it on." I had come a long way for just being out of college for a year (with all that happened in college).

At the Trials you have to race your event a number of times. I had to run the 800m three times in 4 days, which is grueling. The preliminaries were great. I felt fast and ran the 3rd fastest time going into the semi-finals. I was confident. The semi-finals were the day after the preliminaries, and were another story. I felt tired before my race even started and my heat was stacked (meaning that one of the semi-final heats had too many of the fastest girls), and only 4 advanced to the finals.

Needless to say that was the heaviest pushing I've ever been involved in and during the first lap of the race I had someone step on my heel every time I put my foot down, so badly that my hand touched the ground at 200m to keep myself from eating the track, but at 400m I had another big push and by 500m I was out of gas. The jostling comes with the race, what kept me from the finals was my inability to recover from the race the previous day. This was a serious sign that something was wrong, but again I didn't know. Despite all my training and hard work, I didn't make the 2004 Olympics. I just couldn't maintain my speed day after day.

Later the next year, my coach decided to go to the Middle East and train Africans who get paid to run for these Middle Eastern countries. They do this because they don't have enough good athletes themselves. Coach told me I could go over there and train with him, but I wasn't going to go to Africa and I was certainly not going to the Middle East. I had serious concerns about my potential safety.

Coach leaving for the Middle East put a huge strain on our training group. Nobody knew what to do and eventually we all split up and went our separate ways. It was 2005 and we were in the middle of our season. Everyone had to make a decision quickly.

Changing Coaches
and Incredible Stress

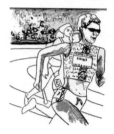

*"Exercise is a dirty word. Every time I hear it,
I wash my mouth out with chocolate."*
– Author Unknown

I found a coach in Orlando, Florida, a black guy with white hair and the craziest looking eyes you've ever seen. He looked like the Grinch who stole Christmas, and was just as much of a character! I had everyone in the running world split on their advice on where I should go. Half said go to this distance group in Oregon and the other half said go to the coach in Orlando. I'm not really a distance runner, that route has never worked for me. I decided to go with the sprinting group in Orlando because that's where I'd had the most success in the past.

The stress of packing all my stuff, slamming it into my car, leaving behind a stray cat I took in (named Binky) whom I loved dearly and finding him a home (where he died soon after, running away from his new family's home), then driving across country, living in the male teammates' apartment for a few weeks while trying to find a house, and going to practice was major stress. And this, my friends, is where the shit hit the fan. My body couldn't deal with it all. The tick bite that occurred nearly two years earlier came back to get me.

I was driving on Highway 10 through the desolate part of Arizona, New Mexico, and West Texas, wondering if I made the right decision. I felt good about it, I was just sad to leave my running group behind because for the first time I was training with people who were not only athletic studs but also good-hearted and a pleasure to train with. (I never felt that way about any other group and still haven't to this day.)

Orlando was way hotter than Tucson. In Tucson you can get in the shade where it's about 20 degrees cooler. Orlando is like South Carolina; there is no relief from the heat. It's just as hot in the shade as it is in the sun because of the 100% humidity. And guess what? Heat kills Lyme.

I was training hard in Orlando. I only had a few months until the US Nationals. I noticed I was having an increasingly hard time recovering between workouts. I also noticed that one day I was on and the next week off. I was extremely fit and doing some world class training. I was ready to BLOW it up on the track, but I ended up imploding instead.

Some days I felt so toxic for some reason, like I couldn't detox the buildup of lactic acid, a phenomenon that occurs in anaerobic training (meaning training so hard your muscles go without oxygen and have to create chemical reactions to create fuel). I would start puking, but not much would come up, just a yellow substance that looked like bile. I thought it was the heat, and by placing ice packs on my groin and neck

I was able to beat back some of that toxicity.

Now looking back, I know exactly what was happening. Being on the track in the summer in Orlando, running hard cooked my insides. Lyme was dying off rapidly, and I was becoming toxic through the stress of running (producing lots of lactic acid) from the heat. But what was really killing me were the neurotoxins being released when the Lyme bacteria died off.

I only had a few weeks to go before the big race. I had trained so hard, and I was amazingly fit. What's interesting is that I was so fit and so sick at the same time! Yes, this is often the story because having the ultimate fitness and being ill can be a very, very thin line.

The day of US Nationals, I felt okay. Perhaps part of it was just being used to down playing illness, which athletes always do. We're so used to pain that we brush off illness blaming it on training. This attitude is the reason why I ignored the bite in the first place. It's why I'm the real reason for my own personal tragedy.

The BOMB

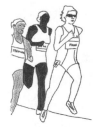

"There are times in everyone's life when something constructive is born out of adversity when things seem so bad that you've got to grab your fate by the shoulders and shake it."
– Author Unknown

High hopes were in the air for my race, the 800m. It's a long sprint although it's a middle distance race. There isn't much pacing: basically, it's an all out sprint for 2 grueling laps. Personally, I love this distance. You have to be a super tough person to run it. In fact, the 800m was banned from the Olympics in 1928 after the women running in it all fell across the finish, where they proceeded to gasp for air and apparently didn't look lady- like. It was finally reintroduced 32 years later in 1960.

I was a little nervous before my race because of my training issues, but I thought, "it's just one race and then it's over." It was a warm day in Southern California, and the sun was just about to go down, then gun went off. The first lap went smoothly. I was in the perfect striking position as we approached 400m, but something didn't quite feel right. By 500m my legs and arms were tingling and getting quite cold and tight. By 600m I was almost in last place, with 200m remaining. Everyone was passing me, and I couldn't do anything about it. My extremities were so cold; I knew something was very wrong. I wanted to stop, but everyone was watching the drama unfold. I finished the race dead last. I was emotionally destroyed, and furthermore I realized I might be physically destroyed as well. My body was like an engine starved of oil and now completely useless.

This experience is enough for any normal person to say never again, but I'm pretty far from being normal and while it was tough growing up, it became an asset as an adult. I was wondering how many times I'd have to get knocked down before I didn't get back up. I didn't see a medic because I knew I was diseased and this was way beyond what a trainer or medic was going to be able to help me with.

I returned to Orlando after the race, packed my stuff and went home to see my parents. I had a health crisis and no idea of what exactly I was going to do. I felt like a huge loser, and all the comforting words in the world couldn't help me. I was defeated beyond belief. A race and a win that should have been mine had fallen through the cracks, again. At this time I had no idea that I wouldn't be racing or even running again for 5 years, I just knew I was really ill.

Immediately upon arriving home, I started scratching the back of my head (the location of the tick bite from a few years prior). My mother took a look at it after she noticed me scratching. She said, "Perry, your bite is back and it looks angry."

What had I gotten myself into? I started looking up tick illnesses online, and I thought "OH MY GOD, I HAVE LYME!" The bite had the Lyme disease bull's eye rash, and during the following months it would grow to cover half of the back of my head.

I needed someone to turn too, someone who had Lyme who could help me. I began contacting groups online and emailing people with blogs (in 2005 there weren't many), and looking hard for some answers. People I talked to were negative, telling me that there was no cure and that I was "screwed." After a few weeks of listening to other Lymies (a term that people with Lyme disease call themselves, which is a very victimizing term for my liking as "Limey" is a derogatory term given to sailors because they would eat limes to keep scurvy away). I quickly realized it was in my best interest to just shut them out completely. No more chatting with other "Lymies." The doom and gloom was just too much and even though I had the same disease, I never wanted to feel like my place was with other sick people. It was a wise choice in retrospect.

Off to See the Expert

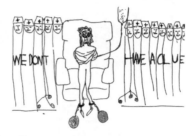

"The deadliest contagion is majority opinion."
– Author Unknown

I got an appointment with a top infectious disease doctor in the Southeast who treats Lyme and HIV. I thought I would just take some drugs and get over it. Boy was I wrong!

My mom and I drove over to Dr. James near Charlotte, North Carolina. I was not feeling very well, but had no idea how much worse it was about to get. Sitting in the waiting room was perhaps the worst part of the visit, as all the people looked like they could keel over at any second. Nobody was cheery. Nobody was perky. Nobody had any hope in their eye. I realized then the severity of the situation. Here I was with HIV patients, and apparently Lyme disease was just as serious.

My appointment with Dr. James was strange, to say the least. I began telling him the situation: when I was bitten, the time that had elapsed, and my athletic feats since the bite. For some reason it didn't register with him. He said to me that he ran the 800m in high school and asked me how fast I ran it. I told him what I ran the past year and he kept saying, "This was before the tick bite." I kept saying, "No, I was already bitten about a year prior." It was pure disbelief. Then, he asked me about taking "roids." My reaction was, "Me, on 'roids?' Ha, ha, you're kidding, right?" I mean, if you saw me in person, there would be no way you'd believe I was juiced. The twins are real (quite big for my frame), no acne, no deep voice, no huge muscles, no beard (or chin hair). I'm a real lady. I told him that I didn't even take Tylenol® so of course I don't take steroids!

Dr. James seems like he is on another planet. Maybe he was down about all the death he sees every day. He ordered a bunch of tests. I went back to get my blood drawn. Before I left, I told him I wanted to get over it 100% and asked him what my chances were. He told me, "We'll do the best we can." But what I heard was: "I have no idea, Perry, but in my medical opinion, you're screwed." It wasn't his words, it was the way he said them.

When you have Lyme, every part of your body hurts and is sensitive to light, sound and touch. Getting pricked with a needle for routine blood work was excruciating enough, but the lady drawing the blood couldn't care less. This enormous lady seemed more interested in squeezing out the last bit of flavor from her gum. I asked her politely to be careful please because I didn't feel well; she smiled like she wasn't listening and jabbed me again, apparently unable to find one of my athletically induced, bulging, blood spurting, surface veins. I was getting heated from this insensitive and unprofessional nurse. It's amazing to me how many people go into the healthcare profession who don't really seem to care about people. I really believe that to be a good health professional, you must really love people.

On July 29, 2005, less than a month since my BOMB OUT at the 2005 USA Track and Field Nationals, Dr. James put me on his arsenal of oral antibiotics.

After a month or so on his poison, my tests came back.

The problem with Lyme testing is that it's not as accurate as one would like. In fact, it's so inaccurate that people who have serious cases of Lyme still don't test positive for it. Because of this symptoms are the determining factor. Of course, having the bull's eye rash helps a lot because then you know you have it, even if a test says you don't. I guess I'm lucky to know I was bitten, and be able to see the bite because it has been my guide this entire time for how well I'm doing. On good days, I would hardly notice it was there. On bad days, it got big and red and angry. If I put salt, or alcohol, or something I thought would kill it (sometimes even oregano oil which has super powerful anti-bacterial properties) it would explode into anger (so, of course, I kept doing it!) I figured if I could make it angry then I was doing something that could kill it. This measurement came in handy as my temperamental bite site helped me figure out what was working and what wasn't.

There are a high percentage of people with Lyme disease who don't know it or don't recall being bitten. It's like a naughty ghost. It's hard enough getting a doctor to test you for Lyme, especially when you can't recall being bitten. Patients are often treated like they are hypochondriacs and dismissed as if it's "all in your head." Heard that one before?

The Tests Come Back

50-50		
Really BAD		
NOT So GooD		
JusT OK		
Close To Really BAD		

*"An expert knows all the answers -
if you ask the right questions."*
– Author Unknown

The worst part of the testing was the lack of explanation provided about the results. This is what really gets me, and doctors do this crap all the time. They don't explain to the patient all of the numbers on that piece of paper. Hey, I paid for it, I want to know everything! Maybe they don't think I'm smart enough …but I really hate to burst their bubble: there's a good chance I am. I eventually did my own research to find out exactly what every single number meant or could possibly mean. Reference ranges for blood work is just a guide. Sometimes the data might be within the reference range, but can still indicate issues.

Dr. James gave me an IgM and IgG Western Blot. This is the most common test used for Lyme disease. IgM tests for recurrent or persistent infections, the IgG tests for recent or active infection. Because these tests are never definitive, it's important to know that many people who have Lyme disease and other tick infections will test negative or indeterminate (equivocal and borderline) because the bacteria is so hard to test for. My tests came back as indeterminate (IND), but I was positive for two bands that were a dead giveaway for someone with Lyme disease. See **Appendix I** for a more detailed explanation of my test results.

Dr. James was sure that I had Lyme disease no matter what the tests said, simply because of my symptoms and my history (and luckily I pulled the deer tick out of the back of my head, no denying that incident). That's why it's so important to go by symptoms, not results. The CDC acknowledges large scale under-reporting, the reasons are (in my own words) first, the testing isn't accurate enough, second, many general practitioners are Lyme illiterate and will not even think to test you for a tick-born illness, (hopefully this will change in the near future) third Lyme, is the "mystery" illness, mimicking many other diseases that are always tested before Lyme is.

I later had the Western Blot done several more times, but I need to tell you that I'm not here to write about all these crazy bands. You can drive yourself nuts by lining up your bands on a timeline and seeing which ones show a positive or a double positive, which ones turn negative or which ones go from negative to IND. Each time you get your results, you hope that they are better, but everybody knows it's not always accurate. International Lyme experts agree that most Lyme antibody tests are made to detect a small percent of the spirochete forms and there are no conventional accepted markers for the majority of intercellular forms which constitute the majority of the Lyme bacterial load[1]. Trust me when I say it's much more important to write down your symptoms in detail and use that as a guide for how far you've come. It will give you satisfaction, and it gives you a better idea of what works and what doesn't when it comes to your overall progress.

I was bitten in North Carolina. There were only 156 cases reported in the state the year I was bitten[2]. The day I was bitten I was in a crowd of people (in the thousands) listening to music. I wasn't the only one "chosen" that day to get bitten. I suspect hundreds of other people were bitten as well. Where there is one tick, there are millions. I wonder how many of those people from that day (at a festival that happens annually) are now sick and have no idea that it's because of a tick bite.

1. "Seronegativity in Lyme borreliosis and Other Spirochetal Infections," http://www.ly-meinfo.net/medical/LDSeronegativity.pdf (accessed January 24th, 2012).; Tom Grier, "Will There Ever Be An Accurate Test for Lyme Disease?" http://www.canlyme.com/flawedtest.html (accessed January 24th, 2012).; Marjorie Tietjen, "Lyme Disease - Misdiagnoses And Medical Dictatorship," http://www.rense.com/general43/kly.htm (accessed January 24th, 2012).
2. CDC, "Reported Lyme disease cases by state, 1999-2009," http://www.cdc.gov/lyme/stats/chartstables/reportedcases_statelocality.html (accessed September 14, 2011).

Chronic Lyme Disease

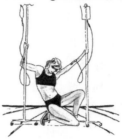

"With willing hearts and skillful hands, the difficult we do at once; the impossible takes a bit longer."
– Author Unknown

L yme is mysterious because only some people who are bitten actually know they were bitten, and are tested quickly and receive antibiotic treatment for a few weeks, recover and get on with their life. Most people don't realize they were bitten, or don't feel sick right away. By the time the disease stars to affect them, years have gone by and it is too late for modern medicine or antibiotics to save the day. But, even people who catch it right away still have problems associated with the tick bite years later, as antibiotic treatment isn't a proven cure for recent infections, nor chronic infections. Sometimes it is successful and many times it isn't.

Chronic Lyme disease is what most people actually have. When symptoms manifest weeks, months or years later they get treatment. It often results when several months of therapy (usually antibiotics) go by and the symptoms are still there even though there is no evidence of the bacteria or a bite. The Bb bacteria are smart. It's usually hiding in other forms unknown to your immune system, trying to evade it as well as the antibiotics. If you have symptoms, you still have it. Many doctors think that chronic means that if the bacteria goes untreated for an extended amount of time, it becomes "almost impossible to get rid of." Research shows Bb being persistent even after antibiotic therapy[1].

The Bb bacteria, the Lyme bacteria, can go into a cyst form if the host's biological terrain is not favorable or it feels like it's being attacked by the immune system, medication or anything that can kill it. In that form it can remain hidden, dormant in the body until conditions change. Then it erupts with a vengeance.

My thoughts on this chronic situation are that symptoms of Lyme can go on because the body's immunological mechanisms have been triggered by the bacteria. I also think that because these "Lyme Literate" doctors aren't giving good detox protocols, the waste from detoxing sulfa-drugs (antibiotics) and trying to detox the neurotoxins from the bacteria dying often accumulates in the body. It causes a super catastrophic phenomena in the body, which is sometimes, if not always, worse than the infection itself. Those people who have "neuroborreliosis" (neurological symptoms) and have very weak immune systems need to focus on detoxing

1. Mursic VP, Wanner G, Reinhardt S, Wilske B, Busch U, Marget W. "Formation and cultivation of Borrelia burgdorferi spheroplast L-form variants." Infection. 1996;24(3):218-26. PubMed.gov,. http://www.ncbi.nlm.nih.gov/pubmed/8811359 (accessed October 12, 2011).

to remove waste and getting rid of inflammation due to the bacteria (or previous inflammation from poor lifestyle habits). To learn more about neurological issues associated with Lyme disease, please see **Appendix II.**

What Else Besides Lyme?

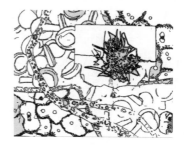

"It just wouldn't be a picnic without the ants."
– Author Unknown

L ike most people with severe autoimmune dysfunction, my blood work was looking bad (indicating a poorly functioning immune system). Besides Lyme, the other parts of a future blood test ordered by another doctor would show that my body was under stress, and was fighting an infection. My lupus panel can back as a weak positive. I would also find out that I had low B12, low carbon dioxide, low carotenoidester, low glutathione…this was like a convention for the severely "deflated." It was incredibly discouraging. I wasn't producing any energy at this time! See a more detailed explanation of my results in **Appendix IIIa**.

One tick can carry tons of nasty bacteria, all with fancy names. My other co-infection tests (for other tick related bacteria) also showed signs of Babesia. Of course with all of the co-infections, it can be confusing, but what I've found is that it doesn't matter. You treat them all the same. Conventional doctors like to focus on the different bacteria and what type of drug can kill each type (even though there is much debate on what works and what doesn't, each patient usually finds themselves becoming a guinea pig for lots of pills with even fancier names than the bacteria they are trying to kill). I would guess doctors were doing the right thing by prescribing antibiotics if they knew an infection was recent and had properly ruled out all other possible health issues. Most people who find out they have Lyme usually do so weeks, months or even years later. By this time the infection is chronic.

Once I went nonconventional, and you'll soon find out what that entails, I realized that to a healthy body these bacterial infections are all the same mess, it's just something that shouldn't be there. More than likely, if you have Lyme disease, you have other types of co-infections. Almost everyone does. Some people have 2 or 3 co-infections, some 4 or 5.

Dr. James wrote up his consultation with me, a one page summary of my history. Dr. James wrote that I "deny any joint aching or muscle aching." This hurt. I get asked by other people who have Lyme disease about the joint inflammation/ arthritic type symptoms. Maybe I did have swelling and aching, but I'm an athlete and am quite used to my muscles hurting. I just couldn't separate the pain of training from the pain of Lyme at that time. I simply thought I was over training. In some aspects, I probably was. You have to walk a fine line between health and ultra fitness to be the best. That's why athletes are so prone to injury, and that's why athletes take "the juice" (steroids).

I'm angry now because Dr. James just put me on a ton of antibiotics. It was like chemo. I felt he ignored all of these other serious issues that could be corrected to help balance my body and fight infection naturally, the way God intended. Had we taken care of those issues first, I may not have almost died from antibiotic therapy. Perhaps, I would have had more of a fighting chance. I am still not sure if it was neglect or just ignorance. What I am sure of is that I'm trying hard to forgive here. To forgive someone you have to acknowledge that person was doing the best they could do with the information they had.

Dr. James gave me this sheet that said take B12, iron, fish oil, flax and aloe vera. Now these are very good supplements, but I had a serious deficiency issue and had already been on B12, so having some nutritional IVs would have been helpful, but I was never given any (unfortunately, many conventional doctors don't believe in many of the integrative therapies). Also, the sheet said to take a probiotic. Probiotics are microorganisms that help quell bad bacteria, fungus and yeasts from growing out of control in the body. Taking antibiotics can cause a huge imbalance to the healthy bacteria in the gut, often causing leaky gut (a term used to describe the damage to the intestinal lining, where the toxins and bacteria in the gut are thought to leak out into the blood stream, causing severe illness in some cases and many autoimmune issues).

With the leaky gut issues to tackle in my near future, taking a probiotic wasn't going to be enough. Major repair had to be done to the gut. Again, I didn't find this out until later.

Not treating these other imbalances in the beginning was my first big mistake. The second was jumping on the drug band wagon and not having a detox protocol. When taking doses of antibiotics, or even following natural treatments that work well on killing Lyme, die-off occurs. Many people talk about the "Herx" reactions or in natural medicine it's sometimes referred to as a "healing reaction." I think of it more as a "detox reaction" because your body is simply over-run with crap it needs to get rid of.

When bacteria dies, it creates neurotoxins that can make you deathly ill. So taking medication (poison) is bad enough, but on top of that is this mass of neurotoxins the body has to dump somehow. If you're sick in the first place, your body isn't processing and eliminating waste well enough, so when you add the stress of neurotoxins floating around, your body goes berserk. Having a plan to detox this die-off is critical. Why didn't my Lyme specialist give me tips, pointers, or some type of plan to help detox me? Is this another bullshit-type-natural medicine idea conventional doctors don't want any part of? If that's the case, they are doing everyone in this country a major disservice.

But the real kicker is that I was tested for testosterone without my knowledge even after I had reassured Dr. James that I was not taking "roids." Now, maybe this is common practice, but I was pretty upset when my next doctor pointed it out to me. The last thing I would do is lie about taking "roids" when I'm trying to be treated for a serious health crisis like Lyme disease. For all of those wondering, it was

51. The normal range is 20-76 for females my age. An entire hormone panel would have been helpful, not just a test for testosterone. Especially since I was picking up the tab for his curiosity.

Dr. James' last comment on the page was the nail in my coffin. It was just his honest opinion of the situation, but reading it felt like a death sentence: "The patient's full recovery is problematic but she is informed of this and is obviously quite upset. However, we cannot guarantee that she will return to the form of a world-class athlete. Nonetheless we are confident that she should receive ongoing pulse oral therapy and hope this will be effective for her."

Boy was this "expert" so wrong about me. I always knew there were answers out there, but I felt like he wrote me off with a stroke of his keyboard on our very first visit. I wasn't looking for a guarantee. I just needed a positive outlook. If my doctor didn't have faith in the situation, how could I? What he didn't write in there is that he told me when leaving the office after that first visit that there was a "good chance" that I would not return to athletics at the level I was on. It was one of the worst days of my life.

Let the Treatment Commence

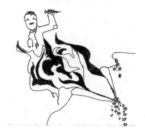

"I don't want the cheese, I just want to get out of the trap."
– Spanish Proverb

I went along with treatment because I didn't know what else to do at this point. This is the basis of Western Medicine – keep the patients ignorant and fearful so they do what you tell them. I didn't know anything more when I left the doctor's office than I had when I arrived, so I was leniently compliant. You could say I was an ignorant fool. So here it comes: Minocycline, Flagyl®, Septra® and Ketek®, Azithromycin (Zithromax®). I felt like a pharmaceutical guinea pig.

"So doc, what are the results from people using these and what can I expect?" No answer. This wasn't very promising, but I went along with it hoping to get rid of these bacteria ASAP and start training again. Plus, at this time I didn't really know of other any options. I couldn't find any good information about what to do for Lyme. All of the information out there was about ticks and the standard protocol for treating Lyme (which I'll be the first to tell you is pretty pathetic). It's poorly researched, and the people getting treatment are basically lab rats. Although, things are getting much better now that more knowledge is being passed and the disease is becoming more and more discussed and success stories like my own are being told.

I picked up my prescriptions and my insurance covered some of it, as well as some of my visit with Dr. James.

I started popping pills all day, every day. My entire day revolved around what I should be taking at what time. Dr. James never gave me antibiotics by IV. Most of the people in his clinic that first day were sitting there with antibiotic IV drips looking like pure death. I guess that's his secret weapon (making sick people sicker). Why would someone who was already terribly ill, and unable to fight off infection, be subjected to an overload of poisons? What I was given was certainly overload and thankfully it didn't kill me, but the ensuing month on this bombing spree created the most dreadful moments of my life. Later on in the journey, I realized that baby doses would have been sufficient especially when I found out that I, like many people, could not detox the type of antibiotics I was given.

I'm in Hell and There's Not a Shred of Hope

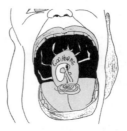

"A healthy body is the guest-chamber of the soul; a sick, its prison."
– Francis Bacon

I was already terribly ill when I first saw Dr. James. Forty-five days later I was in pure hell. I knew I wasn't going back to track and field.

After I started taking my poison, I called my coach and told him the bad news. Coach was disappointed, but no one was as disappointed as me. All I ever wanted to do was to run fast. Coach said something very important to me that stuck with me through the worst of times, making it easier to see the big picture and the light at the end of the tunnel. He said, "God isn't going to take your talent away, Perry. It will always be there. It's just not going to disappear one day." He was so right.

During this ordeal in high school, college and post

collegiate running, dealing with what I guess many athletes go through, I was always trying to hold on to things I thought people were trying to take from me. I've had people try to take my dignity, my pride, my heart, my soul, not to mention material things. But no one can take my medals, my performances, or my talent; these will forever be mine. At this time, everything felt like it was slipping away. My agent didn't even call me back when I told him I had Lyme. I guess he already knew how bad Lyme was, being from the northeastern states and figured I'd never be back.

I was unaware that the darkest hours of my life were about to unfold, and I was going to have to do everything in my power to keep myself from doing something really stupid (as I was losing my mind, not just my body).

The daily pill-popping was revolting. Every time I went to take them, my body screamed "No, don't do it you asshole!" The taste, the smell, the side effects were overwhelming, and every part of my body was telling me not to do it, but I did it anyway. I thought I had too.

After the first few days, I became really sick. I couldn't see straight. My head was constantly spinning. I was falling over. I wanted to puke every hour on the hour. A war was raging inside my body. Bacteria were running scared, and my body was trying hard to balance itself and maintain normal levels of operation.

Before I started taking antibiotics, I was already having a die-off, naturally caused by the heat in Orlando and hard training. I was cooking my insides and that is why I believe I was barfing on the side of the track every time workouts got intense -- I started to burn up from the blazing heat.

As I took the antibiotics, the "healing reactions" occurred in my arm pits mostly. The bacteria were dying off and my lymph nodes were working over-time to remove waste. These red skin rashes appeared over my lymph nodes in my armpits and in my groin. When I took more drugs, these skin rashes grew more intense as well. They hurt to touch. I didn't know what to do about them at this point or how to make them go away. I had no idea I needed to detox myself. Having Herx reactions is not necessarily a good thing. It means your body is full of waste, so killing Lyme on top of that means your body isn't detoxing and the poisons are building up inside. Before taking the drugs, my symptoms included: severe fatigue, skin rashes, the site of the tick bite becoming red, angry and itchy, muscle soreness, sniff neck, photophobia (eyes sensitive to light), sensitivity to sounds, skin hurting to the touch, numbness and tingling in my arms and legs, a sick feeling in stomach, no restful sleep, dry mouth, frequent urination, inability to regulate body temperature and I'm sure there are more I just ignored. When your body is going nuts, there is only so much of it you can actually deal with.

While taking the drugs my symptoms intensified to the nth degree: nonstop vomiting, bed-ridden fatigue and terrible nightmares. What's worse is that many of those symptoms never subsided after my long first round of antibiotics, and subsequently my LAST round.

When I first started my treatment things got really bad, I had to trick my mind into dealing with the situation. For example, there was no relief lying down, none what so ever. I mustered up everything I had to keep trying to do normal daily activities. I drove to my office to work even though I probably shouldn't have been driving. I couldn't see in the sunlight, my shades were never dark enough, and I kept doubling over in pure pain at stoplights. When I was in front of my computer, I couldn't see the screen. Often I would be typing and couldn't see what I was writing.

But feeling bad while keeping busy was much better than feeling bad and lying in bed because I was able to trick my mind into thinking that I could always lie down if I wanted relief (which was total bullshit, although it helped ease the mental situation a little).

Did I Just Snap My Own Neck?

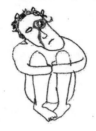

*"Following the path of least resistance is what
makes rivers and men crooked."*
– Author Unknown

One morning, sometime right at the end of the first round of antibiotic treatment, I woke up with a terrible pain in my neck. I had moderate neck pain due to my accident years ago (even though I had a ton of chiropractic care in high school after the incident), but this was something else. I had a sniff neck during my Lyme treatment, but one morning, while getting out of bed I felt a snap in my neck; and suddenly I couldn't move it! It was almost like I had stretched in the wrong way, but I didn't even remember stretching, and my neck felt like it was caught, hung up on something.

I was scared out of my mind because I couldn't move my neck after hearing this loud, awful pop. I was in terrible pain.

It was a Saturday morning, and my mother took me across the street to an emergency clinic.

Now, I'm not the type of person to go the ER unless I seriously suspect something very wrong. Upon arriving at the clinic in my PJ's and walking with my neck cocked to the side in a strange, contorted position, I received many stares from the staff. This was one of those visits that I'll remember for the rest of my life because everyone was so disingenuous, rude and didn't care that I was hurting. It was seriously cruel.

At first they didn't want to see me because I was a new patient, which was bizarre because the clinic was meant for emergency cases (ones that might not be ER type, but nevertheless need medical attention). Then, even though there was basically no one else in the waiting room, they took almost an hour to see me. If that wasn't insulting enough, what with the stares and the whispering (like I couldn't hear), the doctor ended up being completely inept.

I was crying, in terrible pain, needing assistance, and the disgruntled herd of women at the front desk were more interested in their gossip, which included me, than they were in doing their job.

The entire ordeal was traumatizing because I couldn't defend myself (I shouldn't have needed to in a health care facility) against these women who were whispering about me "faking it."

I had some x-rays taken, and the doctor told me (after I mentioned I had Lyme disease), "Oh, you have Lyme disease? I didn't know you could get it down here." My x-rays were fine, nothing broken or hurt. He gave me a prescription for muscle relaxers. A few days later, I was able to move my neck again.

I realize now that I had swollen painful Lymph nodes around my neck area. Because I didn't have a detox protocol and was overloaded with waste, I had toxic fluid around my neck and spine causing the pain and perhaps weakening my neck muscles causing the injury.

Flashing Back

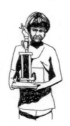

"We learn wisdom from failure much more than from success. We often discover what will do, by finding out what will not do; and probably he who never made a mistake never made a discovery."
– Samuel Smiles

At this point (both before and after the neck incident), I was spending more and more time in bed, staring at the ceiling and crying. I tried not to as it didn't help me one bit; crying just took more out of me, and I didn't have anything to spare. But I lay for hours, sometimes days, crying. The tears just kept coming, falling down my face and pooling at the back of my head, soaking my pillow. It went on like this for too long.

This is when I started to have more intense nightmares. The most vivid was a reoccurring dream that I first had after I left West Point. I dreamt that I walked to the edge of a lake one night and down to the end of a dock where I stepped off the edge. I sank to the bottom like I had weights tied to my feet and no way to get back to the surface. It was like Bud, from the movie Abyss, going all the way down into the unknown and knowing I wouldn't make it back. I ran out of breath as I kept sinking into this dark abyss and when all hope was lost, something stopped me, filled me with one last breath and sent me straight back to the surface. I gasped for breath exhausted. I was saved once more. I'd wake up sweating like I had been swimming and gasping for air; it was startling and deeply unsettling. Even when the dream was over, I still had anxiety from just having it.

Many nights I didn't sleep at all. My body wouldn't allow me to sleep. Maybe because it feared it wouldn't be able to wake back up. Sometimes I would make peace with everything because I didn't think I would be getting up the next morning. Dying in my sleep wouldn't be such a bad way to go, I guessed.

When I wasn't sleeping, my day dreams were like one long flashback of my life up to this point. All I wanted to do was run. I thought about growing up in the country and running around wild, free and often naked. I started running with my dad on the dirt road in front of our house when I was 5. One day I decided to run with him and I've been running ever since.

I didn't go to pre-school, because I didn't want to leave my mom. Kindergarten was dreadful but by first grade I got along with my PE teacher really well. There was a mile course around our playground and I started running a mile every day during recess. In elementary school the only social times were lunch and recess and I had had some confusion about where I was supposed to be. At lunch I sat with the boys because my best friend was there (and it didn't hurt that I looked like one). At this age girls were immersed in their girly-stuff, meanwhile I was pulling the heads off my Barbie's™, face painting them and making pencil toppers. I remember thinking Ken wasn't man enough. To help me get along, I continued to eat with the boys and started to run during recess.

All I had to do was run 4 laps, and I earned a certificate for my achievement. I was hooked. In fact, I ran every single day while my friends hung out and waited for me to finish. Sometimes I would have a cheering squad. Sometimes other boys challenged me, but their half-hearted attempts always failed. It was customary for my PE teacher to watch everyone run a mile so that he/she could get their certificate, but she was so bored watching my easy win every day that she just told me to come by her office to get my certificate. Sometimes she just left one outside her office, already signed. Eventually she had me just place a check on a piece of paper for each day I ran the mile, and at the end of the week, she tallied it up and gave me my certificates once she had time to get them together. To my sweet surprise she gave me a huge certificate to commemorate my 100th mile, then 200th, then 300th, then 400th, then 500th. I wallpapered my bedroom with them.

Remembering the past kept me thinking about how important it was for someone like me to get healthy again and to keep going. I was happy and free then; I wanted to make it back to that place. I feared the life I would have if I didn't.

Have I Gone Completely Nuts?

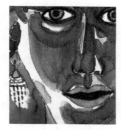

"Madness takes its toll. Please have exact change."
– Author Unknown

A few years ago a woman lived with a chimp for a long time. It was big news when the chimp attacked her and "ripped her face off[1]." It was also big news when a teenage boy went into his church and shot his pastor in Tennessee[2]. In 2005 FSU benched their quarterback[3]. Local police found him lying in the street and saying he was God[4]. What do these stories have in common? If I didn't

1. Andy Newman, Anahad O'Connor, "Woman Mauled by Chimp Is Still in Critical Condition," http://www.nytimes.com/2009/02/18/nyregion/18chimp.html (accessed January 24th, 2012).

2. CNN Justice, "Church shooting suspect planned 'day of death,' prosecutor says," http://articles.cnn.com/2009-03-10/justice/church.shooting_1_keith-melton-illinois-state-police-director-rev-fred-winters/2?_s=PM:CRIME (accessed January 24th, 2012).

3. Miranda Hitti, "Lyme Disease Benches FSU Football Quarterback," Fox News, July 11, 2005, http://www.foxnews.com/story/0,2933,162186,00.html (accessed October 15, 2011).

4. Jill Chandler,"Former FSU QB Arrested Again," WCTV.TV, http://www.wctv.tv/home/headlines/Former_FSU_QB_Arrested_Again_117964814.html (accessed October28 2011).

know about Lyme disease, I would probably say LSD. The chimp and the Tennessee boy were being treated for Lyme disease and the quarterback was suffering from the effects of Lyme disease. Only in the story about the quarterback did the reporting really emphasize the Lyme connection.

Fortunately I was rational enough to not go on a killing spree, but I had crossed over into that world of depression shortly after getting this first round of treatment with high doses of antibiotics. One of the few reliefs I got mentally was visiting a local forestry park. Two service roads and miles of bike trails on the outskirts of town was a place I began to frequent. I didn't go to exercise. I went to sit in the leaves, sometimes for hours on end. I would easily be there all morning, afternoon and sometimes evening without even realizing how long I was gone for.

During that hellish time where I spent so much time in bed, my cat Zippy (she enjoyed running fast, imagine that) provided a lot of comfort. Zippy was a tiny, skinny little black cat that my sister found in Charleston sitting on top of her car tire during a rain storm. Someone had put a box of cats out in the middle of the road and Zippy made her way to my sister's car, where she was retrieved sitting on the tire completely soaked. She became my pet and had been with me for years before I became sick. It's bizarre the close relationships people can have with their pets, as if they can communicate with each other in a glance. Zippy had always provided so much comfort, if there were ever a soul mate pet, Zippy was it. She loved to run, was intelligent and could stand her ground.

One day my parent's neighbors were complaining about a dead odor coming from underneath their deck. It was

Zippy and she was dead. Her body had already decomposed. Her death challenged me as I was tip toeing on the edge on insanity already. My mind was already half way to hell and three sheets to the wind due to the massive drugs I was taking. I immediately remembered that the rental house on the end of the street had a truck parked in their driveway Friday afternoon and there were pesticides in the back. I was furious and my anger was close to being uncontrollable.

After doing a little digging, I found out they had sprayed for "tree roaches" and sprayed mulch and put it all over the ground. Several birds and squirrels had died as well. The company who oversaw the property wouldn't give me any straight answers. Zippy died a few feet from where the mulch was put down. (Pesticides and herbicides are powerful neurotoxins and are carcinogens that can make people very ill. They are fat soluble, which means they can stay in the body for a lifetime and when concentrations are high enough they can cause life threatening illness. Alternatives should always be used.).

My anger was intense and it took me months to talk myself out of doing something terrible to everyone I felt was responsible. I was actually plotting to commit arson at this point. I had a fantastic plan to get even and the antibiotics were directing my mind beyond a reasonable state. I daydreamed of bringing everyone's house down on top of them. I only knew of one person who killed someone. I went to school with this boy who lived in a trailer and he killed his dad and step mom with a shotgun one night because they wouldn't let him go the skating rink. He then buried them in a shallow grave right behind the house and went to school the next day.

I knew I wasn't like that kid, but I couldn't stop the rage.

My crazies were literally medically induced. I wasn't crazy before I started popping pills, even with Lyme running rampant. But now, I was completely out of my mind from the emotional stress, medications and the Lyme disease. I was close to hurting myself or someone else.

During the antibiotic therapy, things went downhill fast. My body was not my own. I didn't have any control over it anymore. I still tried to use my mind to heal, but things got so bad that every day I constantly had to push back these penetrating thoughts of suicide. I didn't want to tell my parents because I didn't want them to know how far off the deep end I was. I wanted to tell my mother to commit me so badly on certain days when I felt like I had no control at all. I thought perhaps we could borrow a straight jacket for a few days or even hours, until the crazies passed. I struggled with the idea of asking for help because I didn't want anyone to know how bad off I really was. I was embarrassed.

I was at rock bottom and stayed there for months even after the antibiotic treatment was over. Unknown to me, my best friend was getting ready to kill himself at this very same time. I wouldn't find out until a year later that he did it. When my mom found out, she decided to keep it from me because I wasn't healthy enough to handle the information.

Two months after my first appointment, I got a call from Dr. James' office. I had called many times but each time I got a different person on the phone. It was beyond frustrating. Finally a nurse practitioner under Dr. James called me back. I told her how worried I was about the treatment and how bad things were. I voiced my concern about not being able to run again if I continued the treatment, and to my surprise she told me that I shouldn't worry and that I could take a few months off to go back to running and training. Then I could have another treatment.

Her audacity was too much too describe. I was basically bed ridden, but this nurse practitioner was telling me that I could go back to running if I wanted too. That was hilarious! I couldn't even walk without struggling. This was when I realized that these people really didn't know what they were doing and that they really didn't understand. I never went back. In fact, I never called back. I basically "fired" one of the top Lyme disease specialists in the country. To be honest, it was scary, but it also felt really good. I was taking control again.

Keep Believing

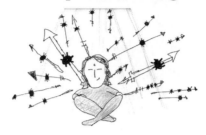

"There are seasons in human affairs, when new depths seem to be broken up in the soul, when new wants are unfolded in multitudes, and a new undefined good is thirsted for. There are periods when to dare, is the highest wisdom."
– William Ellery Channing

Even though I was half crazy at this point, taking matters into my own hands helped me refocus. Now I had a mission to get myself better and there was no time to feel sorry for myself. I held the crazies off and moved forward.

I had hope, but it was buried deep down inside. The sanity issue continued to come and go. On good days, most of my day dreaming was of running. One night, a year into my alternative treatments, I had the most amazing dream. I was running in a race and for every step I took, my competition had to take two. I easily defeated them. I ran smoothly, effortlessly, like I was barely touching the ground. It's impossible to fully describe the sensation, but some of my best races had felt just like this. Was I dreaming about my own future? Maybe I was just reaching out to it through my subconscious, telling my body that I would be back. Somewhere deep down inside I had already made the turning point, I had set my mind to achieve a full recovery.

Even though I was terribly ill, there was a tiny spark deep down inside that just wouldn't be extinguished. Nobody could take this spark away, it remained untouched. It's the reason that even when there was nothing to be hopeful for I knew I would recover completely.

On the surface it was a different story. People don't realize this, but we talk to ourselves daily. The mental chatter in my head was often negative, but I worked hard to shut it up. Every time I caught myself saying "I'm never going to get over this," I would silence it. It's easy to let these negative thoughts dominate when there is absolutely no hope in sight. Especially when you're sick and there are no visible signs of help or relief.

The stress of thinking about the career I had lost was overwhelming. It produced such negative effects that I simply had to let the idea of running go. One day, I just stopped thinking about it. I shut it off. I tuned it out. My goal became to live a normal life again because the thought of going back to running was so far-fetched.

Trying a New Way with Integrative Medical Treatments

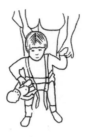

"The best way out is always through."
– A Servant to Servants (1914) Robert Frost

N ow that I knew I wasn't going back under the care of Dr. James, I started researching my options and hoping I could find a way to cure myself. One of my father's clients had a heart condition and was trying to find a cure without having to go under the knife. When he heard about my condition, he told my parents that I might want to go see this lady doctor not too far from my home. I was ready to try anything, so, I went.

Dr. Rachel had a practice in a tiny town on the border between North Carolina and South Carolina, where the foothills reach the Blue Ridge Mountains. As an MD, she treats patients as naturally as possible, so she is really an Integrative Medical Doctor because she incorporates many treatments and philosophies from NDs (Naturopathic Doctors). I went to Dr. Rachel because I knew I had to pump my system up fast and in a very serious way. I was on the cusp, believing I'd be in the ER any day. I started seeing Dr. Rachel in late 2005.

Dr. Rachel was great, very sincere and caring. She also wasn't afraid to say "I don't know." She was involved with medical academia so if she didn't know something, she would try her best to help me figure it out.

Dr. Rachel gave me another Western Blot for IgM and IgG tests. She also tested my levels of hormones, minerals, vitamins, electrolytes and eventually a liver enzyme test to determine my body's ability to detox different substances. When the Western Blot test came back, the IgM results had barely changed. Remember, this tests the persistent infection. It was a hair better, because one band went from IND to Negative. But my overall results were still IND (indeterminate). My IgG results went from IND to Negative, probably because one of the major Tell-All bands, 23 kDa, went from positive to IND. Because of the unreliability of these tests, the results weren't very significant.

Dr. Rachel also tested me for Epstein-Barr virus (EBV) again. When you have something like Lyme, prior illnesses can be activated, especially ones that your body never shakes, the ones you just cope with and move on. My EBV was strongly activated again because of the Lyme. A score over 19 is positive; my IgG Nuclear Antigen (recent or chronic infection activity) was 189. Some of my inexplicable fatigue was coming from this recurring virus.

I also had dysautonomia, a broad term used to describe a nervous system problem. Vasovagal is a type of dysautonomia, which, I was told by a previous doctor there was no cure for and that it was common among athletes because of having a low heart rate and low blood pressure. Having this condition is actually extremely dangerous and I believe that some well known runners have died not because of "natural causes" but because of not having the proper electrolyte balance. Extreme exercise on a body that is not balanced can kill anyone.

Some people with this condition have it so bad that they actually pass out when standing up quickly, like me, or they see visual "snow". At this time, I had no idea how to cure it, but I did by the end of my Lyme recovery.

Urine Loading Test and TSH

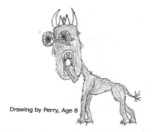

Drawing by Perry, Age 8

*"In order to change we must be sick and
tired of being sick and tired."*
– Author Unknown

urine loading test for iodine came back and showed that I had low iodine. Low iodine means no "gas" in the "gas tank." I was given an iodine supplement. I also had my thyroid checked, and although it came back within reference range, I'm here to tell you that even if your numbers are within range, you can still have a thyroid dysfunction. A doctor who is specifically looking for thyroid dysfunction will pay extra attention to slight nuances in the results, even when they are in reference range. Some doctors will treat thyroid problems (with results in the reference range) in the presence of elevated antibodies (another test). It's very important to make sure your thyroid is functioning properly, as this gland makes and stores the hormones that regulate heart rate, blood pressure, metabolism and body temperature, to name a few.

A test for hormones T3, T4, thyroid-stimulating hormone (TSH) and a free thyroxine index were given. Having an illness like Lyme can certainly hurt your thyroid's ability to do its job. I believe many people may have a problem before they even get Lyme, so it's imperative that it's checked. See **Appendix IV** for more information on thyroid function and indications of thyroid dysfunction.

My T4 was on the low end and my TSH at this time was 1.367 (within reference range, which is .350 to 5.500, but the new standard has a narrower range of .3 to 3.00). My mother was tested for thyroid issues and was having all the symptoms of a hypothyroid (weight gain, tiredness, dry skin, constipation and feeling of being too cold or too hot). Her doctor told her she didn't have a problem. After I saw her test, I told her to go ask him for Armour® (a natural from of thyroid hormone from a desiccated thyroid). She went back, schmoozed him and got it. He gave her the prescription, and with a small dose of Amour in the morning and my suggestion of a thyroid building supplement at night, she felt a huge relief from her fatigue.

Even people with seemingly normal TSH like mine can have hypothyroidism. I surely didn't fit the profile for it at this time, but I did about a year later when I was tested again, because my T4 was so low I suspected an issue with my thyroid. Because of my iodine test, I simply replenished my iodine levels to try to regulate the issue at this time (Iodoral® was the chosen supplement). Even though this put much needed iodine back into my body, it still did not completely fix the problem. My thyroid function wasn't really looked at until a year or so later by another doctor. I believe it could have been skewed naturally from training hard, sweating out minerals for so long, and then, of course not eating foods that were iodine rich. The other issue is that the Lyme was simply causing havoc, creating my thyroid problem.

ASI: Adrenal Stress Index

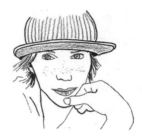

*"While we may not be able to control all that happens to us,
we can control what happens inside us."*
– Ben Franklin

A few other tests later on revealed adrenal stress issues. The adrenals make hormones (such as cortisol, estrogen, progesterone, steroids, cortisone and other chemicals such as adrenalin, epinephrine, norepinephrine, and dopamine) and are the glands that help you fight stress. I believe they are the first things to go in most people who have severe stress or illness. My Adrenal Stress Index™ (ASI) test found that my cortisol was depressed in the morning and elevated at midnight. So I was basically exhausted in the morning and couldn't sleep at night. It takes months to rebuild adrenal glands and their functions once they are shot, but it can be done!

For my adrenals I started taking licorice extract in the

morning to jump-start them. I was given this by a kinesiologist years earlier, and it works quite well (I took it because I was training so hard, and my adrenals were taking a hit). I also started to take a product that had a blend of adaptogens and nutrients that support adrenal function. Adaptogens are substances, usually herbal in nature, that help the body resist the effects of stress. See **Appendix V** about bio-identical hormones and more information on adrenal exhaustion.

I was also given phosphorylated serine (an adaptogen for adrenal support) to help me regulate my cortisol issue naturally. I ended up taking this product twice about 3 months apart. However, I was still having a problem sleeping several months later, even though I was doing much better.

Genomic Test

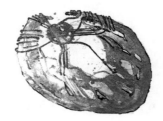

"The doctor of the future will give no medicine, but will instruct his patient in the care of the human frame, in diet and in the cause and prevention of disease."
– Thomas Edison

I was finding out the extent of my metabolic and physiological problems which was a huge downer. I had adrenal problems, a thyroid issue, a hormone issue, and my EBV was reactivated. I had tick bacteria still causing havoc and my genomic test came back positive for a liver detoxing problem. (See **Appendix VI** for information on the test and how my results were interpreted.) This test is called the DetoxiGenomic™ Profile by Genova Diagnostics®. It identifies genetic variations that may affect someone's ability to detoxify specific toxins, medications and foods. There are two phases for the human body to detox.

Phase 1 is the first-line defense, enzymes in the liver help change the structure of the toxin to make it easier to excrete.

There are different enzymes that are responsible for different types of toxins. Medications all have to be broken down by these enzymes and when these specific enzymes are not fully functional (in many people they aren't), these toxins literally back up and can make someone very ill, the same medications that are suppose to make us better make these people sick.

Phase 2 is when the toxin is acted on again by the body adding water-soluble molecules to it. Phase 1 is the reactive phase, and Phase 2 is the eliminations (or dumping) phase.

Some toxins to note are pollution, pesticides, herbicides, pharmaceutical drugs and charbroiled foods. (That's right you might want to stop grilling your food!)

The testing concluded I had several variations in genes that cause my liver not to detox completely like nature intended. It may sound like I'm a mutant, but having variations in genes is how nature works. Most people, if not all, have some variations in their genes responsible for detoxing substances.

People with Lyme disease often describe the same feelings I had about feeling toxic and overburdened. If someone has a hard time dumping the waste from Lyme disease, their bodies may be working overtime not only to detox bacteria but also other substances. Every time I cleaned the bathroom with bleach, glass cleaner, and sink cleaner they were absorbed into my skin or I inhaled them. Everything you put on our skin, you absorb into your bloodstream. After knowing this, I banned all cleaning products with harsh chemicals in them. I went into my bathroom and got rid of any shampoos, toothpaste, face cream, sunscreen, makeup, you name it... they all have toxic chemicals in them that I would eventually have to detox.

I've read that a woman who wears makeup every day will absorb 5 lbs of chemicals each year. Shampoos and lotions contain propylene glycol, an ingredient in anti-freeze (which is super toxic). Sodium Laurel Sulfate (SLS) is carcinogenic and is in damn near everything in your bathroom.

I've been free of these household hazards and toxins for almost three years, and I look good and feel good. I've found many alternatives that work just as well and aren't a hazard to my health. With Lyme disease, to truly heal, you must get rid of all the unnecessary problems. For me, changing this lifestyle issue was just another thing that needed to be done to solve my health problem.

IV Vitamin C

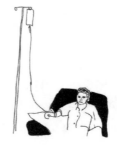

*"Start by doing what's necessary; then do what's possible;
and suddenly you are doing the impossible."*
– Francis of Assisi

One of the best treatments from Dr. Rachel was the IV vitamin C (see **Appendix VII** on how this works and **Appendix 2-III** for an in depth review of how IV vitamin C works various medical conditions by vitamin C researcher and proponent, Dr. Levy). There is a lot of debate on whether this works, but I'm here to tell you it does! This is why I decided to go to her in the first place. I really wanted to try this treatment out. People are using it for all types of reasons from bacterial diseases to cancer. It just makes people feel great! This treatment is good for detoxifying chemicals, strengthening organs, and cleansing the liver.

After the first day of getting IV vitamin C, which was done on my second visit, I was able to walk up the stairs in my house for the first time since seeing Dr. James, the tick doctor. I had strength in my legs again. I was hooked.

I got this IV at Dr. Rachel's office once or twice a week getting my 3-hr drip, a 75g vitamin C treatment. Some people get up to 100g; a urine test is needed to find out what your amount is because sometimes a 100g treatment is worthless because your body can handle only 60g, so 40g goes to waste. Everyone's saturation level is different and one should know that taking vitamin C by IV is not the same as taking it orally. IV vitamin C produces substantially higher vitamin C concentrations in the blood.

I was also taking a form of beta-glucan called "Tsi-Ahga" at this time (see **Appendix VIII** for more information on this specific type). It targets inflammation associated with infection. It is naturally anti-microbial and helps prevent and treat many different bacterial, fungal and parasitic infections. As a natural immune enhancer and antioxidant, it can actually increase lymphocyte production. Lymphocytes are a type of white blood cell that carries out the majority of the activities of the immune system.

At the end of my 75g IV vitamin C treatment, a B complex injection was added to the bag. I believe the treatment was extremely helpful in boosting my own immune system and helping me flush out some of the waste from the die-off. I had about 56 treatments of IV vitamin C from the end of 2005 to the end of 2006. What's interesting is that I had just as many Herx reactions as I did when I took the conventional approach with antibiotics.

Herxing is not usually considered a good thing, but I felt like it was a positive thing because I wasn't taking anything harmful and was apparently still having die-off, which was strengthening my belief that a full recovery could be had without taking medications. My theory after this experience is that you can kill off pathogens without having Herx reactions if your body can properly detox well enough.

Maybe the vitamin C was effective in killing off the Lyme. People at this clinic were feeling good, and many of these people had just as serious issues as the people in Dr. James' clinic. One day a girl, 14, came in who had Lyme disease, sat beside me in a recliner getting treatment. I spoke with her briefly, but she seemed to tune me out. This girl was hopeless, but I was trying to get her to understand that it would work out because I was realizing that there was light at the end of the tunnel. My spirits were lifted, and I was finally getting over the dead feeling I had had since 2005.

Triple Whammy

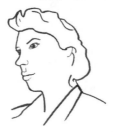

"Never be afraid to try something new.
Remember, amateurs built the ark;
professionals built the Titanic."
– Anonymous

While I was doing IV vitamin C, I decided to include a salt and C protocol (a method of taking high oral doses of vitamin C with high doses of salt). I also included garlic pills in this regimen. My dad said that most soldiers came back from Vietnam without strange parasites because they were taking salt tablets. Imagine the water those soldiers must have been wading through and drinking; it's hard to believe more of them didn't get sick with some type of "third world cootie." So I decided to try the protocol with my IV vitamin C. I took vitamin C orally along with high doses of salt to "pickle" my insides and kill the bacteria. I also took garlic (in no real protocol fashion) after researching its excellent activity against a wide range of bacteria and fungal infections. To view more information on a study done on stabilized allicin (one of the active chemicals in garlic), please visit: *www.TheTickSlayer.com/allicin*

When I did this, I actually had increased Herx reactions although this kitchen treatment made me feel bad from eating all that salt. I didn't take conventional salt tablets because they are heavily processed. So I measured my own high quality Himalayan mineral salt instead. Mineral salt has a much lower concentration of sodium than regular table salt (Sodium Chloride) so it is easier on your body as well. To get the scoop on the differences in salt and how Himalayan salt is a good choice for everyone, go to *www.TheTickSlayer.com/salt*.

One to four grams of vitamin C (just below bowel tolerance because you will get diarrhea from taking large amounts of vitamin C) should be taken with the salt. It should be noted that the type of vitamin C ingested should be a form of calcium ascorbate, or sodium ascorbate, go to *www. TheTickSlayer.com/vitc*, to get information on these special types of vitamin C. I did this for several weeks, stopped and did it again until there were no signs of die-off, vomiting, Herx marks on my skin, or bad body odor. I went through 3 weeks of taking this combo in less than a two month time span.

Time to Move on Again

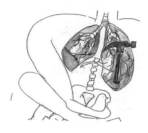

"Resolve says, 'I will'. The man says, 'I will climb this mountain. They told me it is too high, too far, to step, too rocky, and too difficult. But it's my mountain. I will climb it. You will soon see me waving from the top or dead on the side from trying.'"
– Jim Rohn[1]

I knew something was still amiss. But I had no idea what it was. Getting IV vitamin C and taking those new natureceuticals was helping, but something was still not quite right. I could tell. I just didn't know if it was Lyme or not.

Dr. Rachel works with a Chinese Medicine Doctor, who I'll call Dr. Cady. This is an interesting situation because most MD's would never give any credence to this type of medicine. I was totally going to try it!

Dr. Cady is pretty amazing. She had studied in China, and her clinic looked like a 16th century Chinese medicine shop.

1. Quote from Jim Rohn, America's Foremost Business Philosopher, reprinted with permission from Jim Rohn International ©2011.

She had herbs from the floor to the ceiling, neatly arranged and straight across the sea from the Red Land. Dr. Cady was probably one of the most compassionate practitioners I've come across to this day. She understood what it meant to have a bedside manner as a health care professional and she really cared about her patients. She and Dr. Rachel conferenced to figure out what to do with me next. I proceeded to go to Dr. Cady more and more and Dr. Rachel less and less. My mother was still driving me at this point even though I could now drive; it was more of a struggle than it should have been for longer trips, but never-the-less it was progress.

Each visit I would talk to Dr. Cady, show her my health calendar, let her do some strange pulse reading and testing like showing her my tongue. She helped me work through emotional issues as well. What's interesting is that she brought up the fact that "Herxing" was really "healing" reactions and that before this all was over, I might relive some of the worst tragedies I had experienced.

She said sometimes recovering from major illness makes someone release all of their pent-up emotional poison. I thought, *me have emotional issues? No way!* Oh, but she was so right. What's even freakier is that this woman was right about everything! She had a profound sense of intuition and knew what I was going to say before I said it, and knew how I felt before I explained it. Obviously not all Chinese medicine doctors are like this. I think that I found a real gem and that lady was on top of her game.

Dr. Cady is not anyone you'd likely forget. She had short hair except for this one long braided rat tail that stretched a good foot or more down her back. I kept staring at it on my first visit and wondered what that was all about. I think Chinese monks often have this rat tail, (called a "queue") and it's a serious symbol (a hairstyle imposed on the Han Chinese by the Manchu/Qing dynasty); however, you usually expect to see "rat tails" hanging out of a trucker's hat where I'm from, which is an indication of how much someone likes to party.

I had acupuncture (see **Appendix IX** about how acupuncture works) that hurt like hell every time I went. Since I was already sensitive because of the Lyme, my skin ached. But I was doing much better with these treatments and a few months later under Dr. Cady, I was actually driving to my appointments myself. Dr. Cady was trying to treat me for everything that she felt was a problem and interestingly enough her investigative work up each time I went to visit was slightly different. Having a "damp liver" was something that was always a problem; however, I also had issues with my kidneys and other organs that were struggling due to the Lyme. Each time I went I felt more and more relief, like I was being freed up emotionally and physically and I was gaining energy.

Dr. Cady also burned a Chinese "moxa" herb on my belly and I would leave her office smelling like I just smoked a big doobie. This treatment is called "moxibustion" and is used to stimulate and warm acupuncture points and dispel dampness. It is used heavily on people with HIV (or other serious autoimmune disorders) because they are said to have low body energy, a white-coated tongue and poor digestion (indicative of what they call "dampness"). Moxibustion in acupuncture has also been used to correct breeched babies successfully in studies. There are many applications for this treatment.

Dr. Cady would sometimes place it on the end of needles and burn it. Then I would lie down with all of these needles in my body, some giving me terrible pain (like having electricity shock you in certain areas) and stare at the ceiling while I was covered in moxa smoke.

Her clinic was in a Victorian house and it felt relaxed and kind of like being at home. Some visits she would ask me questions about things I didn't want to talk about, but I knew I had to let myself talk about them. She had me working through a lot of things, and most treatments had me lying on the table crying, not in pain but because I was reliving emotional issues and trying so hard to just let it all go.

I sometimes went to Dr. Rachel for IV vitamin C before I headed home. It became a good combination therapy.

Am I Going to Die?

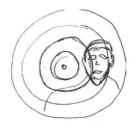

*"You may not realize it when it happens, but a
kick in the teeth may be the best thing in
the world for you."*
– Walt Disney

O ne day Dr. Cady said I was going to get really sick before I got better. I kept thinking, sicker than I've been? I was worried because I didn't want to go back to my antibiotic days. Maybe she knew I was getting ready to release the mother lode of anger, or it was like when a fever finally breaks. Is this what happens with Lyme? Does it reach a tipping point when your body finally takes control after a massive struggle? Do you really have to go to rock bottom to move on? Dr. Cady just reassured me that I was on the right path and that what was coming had to come and I had to go through it to get to the other side.

And then it happened.

My sister complained of a stomach bug one day. She was

sick for a few hours, and apparently my dad got it the next day. He was sick for a little longer, and it looked like it was a bit of a "toilet clinger" type illness, one where you sit on the can (or hang on to "the can") for a period of time in awful pain. I've had these before. I've eaten at a restaurant, and then WHAM, at 2 a.m. I'm running to the bathroom. These food-borne illnesses aren't contagious, but maybe my dad and sister were passing some kind of stomach flu to each other.

I stayed clear of both of them. I was pretty much hibernating those days anyway, trying to rebuild my strength, but I wasn't completely dead anymore. At 8 p.m. one night, the storm blew in.

Sitting in my bed, I realized I was feeling really ill. Then I started making repeated trips to the bathroom. By 9:30 p.m. I was in extreme pain, and it was just intensifying, which was strange because these stomach bugs don't usually happen this way. I thought I was going to die around 11 p.m. This was like nothing I'd ever experienced before, and to this day I have no idea what happened. (While in Bolivia training for the 2004 Olympic Trails, I drank some bad water and was wrecked with pain. I was sweating, squirming around in my bed, screaming. Then, after some medical folk came into our house and gave me a tranquilizer in the butt and some antibiotics, I began peeing out this dead white stuff. Long story short, this was way worse.)

My mother was sitting there in a chair in the hall asking me if I should go to the ER. What was the ER going to do with this mystery illness? Give me a tranq in the butt like an Andean Cat? (I had already been on that run in Bolivia) Give me some antibiotics? Would antibiotics even help this situation? Was it Lyme? It surely wasn't anything I ate, that I knew for sure.

The pain was unbearable, and I started making my way to the bathroom, but unlike my dad who was sitting on the can, I was throwing up into the can. But, I wasn't throwing up anything I had eaten. It was a yellow sludge that looked like bile. I couldn't get enough of it out. I tried desperately to force it out. I was burning hot, so I took all my clothes off. Then I proceeded to freeze to death, so I ran a hot bath and jumped in it.

I remember some years ago while in Tucson I met a guy who had cerebral palsy, he was an avid biker, riding 100 miles in a single day. He told me it was the only way to keep his disease under control. While visiting his house, I remember seeing a tub filled with water that he constantly kept hot. He would jump in when the pain was too excruciating. He took tons of pain meds, but the hot water seemed to keep his muscles from twisting and contorting out of control. I was now in the same situation as my muscles were twisting and knotting themselves.

There was a battle in my body, and I lost control of any kind of functions until 7 a.m. the next morning. At 1 a.m. that night the pain was so bad, I was getting into the hot water more and more often, but then would suddenly become so overheated that I thought I was going to pass out. I would jump out quickly and lay on the hard wood floor naked, yelling obscenities. I'm not the type of person to make a stink about things, and I felt so bad for keeping my mother up, but I couldn't control the cussing, the pain, or the emotions. I was being invaded, and my body was fighting desperately to keep itself together.

About 3 a.m. I was so delirious I started cussing at the Lyme. I hugged the toilet bowl and began to develop a form of bacteria induced Tourette's. Then I would let go with blood curdling screams (and occasional laughter). As I came out of the bathroom, crawling on the floor, soaking wet from my hot bath, I was surrounded by my parents' cats who looked like they were trying to get over their fear of the situation to come and help me. All of them stared at me like they were terrified and that they knew I was somehow possessed by something. If they could talk, they would have been asking me, "What can we do? Tell us damnit!"

That night was the craziest I've ever had in my life. It even trumped the night that I got alcohol poisoning and kept myself awake because I feared dying on my own vomit in the middle of the night (I was in college and pretty pissed off about my running situation, so I decided to let loose in a very bad way). It trumped the worst night of sickness brought on by my first round of antibiotic treatment for the Lyme. It was the sickest I had ever been, or ever would be again.

It took me about a week to return to normal from the ordeal, and afterwards I just kept getting better, quicker and with more ease. I still don't know how Dr. Cady knew that was going to happen. When I told her later about it, she just said "Oh good," and then changed the herbs she was giving me. Part of her therapy was giving me herbs, a strange mix consisting of all types of things. I couldn't begin to tell you what was in them and it's customary for me to pump someone for information, but I was going through so much that I couldn't focus and just went with the flow. For some time Dr. Cady made me eat only cooked vegetables because apparently I was too sick to eat anything else; eating foods that are tough to digest can take away the energy that the body needs to focus on healing.

Dr. Cady told me that I had to start exercising again. I dreaded those words because even walking still hurt. She said 10 minutes a day, 3 times a day. It seemed like it would be the hardest thing ever, and at first it was. I would get up in the morning and start walking in my pajamas. I didn't care what anyone thought. I walked up and down the street trying to get my 10 minutes in. I knew it was important to keep going physically, so I did.

Even under Dr. Cady's care I still knew that there was still something not quite right, but I had made remarkable progress. I was actually living quite normally again after a few months of this double treatment from both doctors.

Still Working

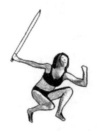

*"Our greatest glory is not in never failing, but in
rising up every time we fail."*
– Ralph Waldo Emerson

E ven though I was ill, I still had to work. In fact, it was
good that I did. I think too many people throw in the
towel and go straight to the couch. People who do
that are sending the wrong signals to their bodies. I worked
despite my annoying neurological and physiological issues. I
was on a business trip to Chicago in the winter and had just
finished working as an apprentice for marketing guru who had
millionaire clients in every corner of the United States and in
other countries. He was putting on a marketing conference.
Nobody, not even the guy I was working for, knew how ill I
really was. I didn't tell anyone.

At these types of events the air conditioning is kept really
low (to keep people awake) and you freeze if you're not eating

whale blubber or wearing a seal skin coat. I couldn't control my body temperature during the event. I went from hot to freezing cold. Still it was not as bad as that "night from hell", but it was enough to make my muscles shake uncontrollably. I had on a nice suit and during breaks I'd go back to my hotel room, take all my clothes off and get in the tub filled with hot water. It was the only way I could get relief without taking pills of some sort. My muscles were already twisted in knots, but being cold exacerbated the problem. I did this the entire conference and nobody, not even my colleagues knew that I was ill. I just put on a big smile and kept going.

A few months after the conference, I flew to Boston for business. The final destination was Martha's Vineyard. The lady I was meeting told me to bring a jacket. She should have said bring a coat, gloves, hat and tights. It was April and while April is warm and hot in the South, it's damn near freezing in Martha's Vineyard. I spent the entire weekend shivering and was in terrible neuromuscular pain and had to tell them what exactly was wrong with me. Martha's Vineyard has one of the highest incidences of Lyme disease, so they knew all about it.

Apparently people in the north are far more familiar with Lyme disease, especially on the island of Martha's Vineyard. While on the ferry over there, I saw deer swimming to the island. My host explained that the deer might not be able to see the island but their instincts helped them to travel back and forth through the ocean and that the island is full of Lyme ticks. Watching the deer that day, looking at the patterns of how Lyme disease actually spread, made me realize the real truth of the situation and about the germ labs off the coast of New York.

Plum Island is a federal germ facility where the creation of Lyme disease is said to have originated as part of germ warfare during World War II. The facility sits off the eastern tip of Long Island's North Fork and if you took a good look at where the Lyme disease cases are and their migration across the US, you'll see that they are stemming from Plum Island.

Hot Car Sauna

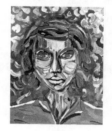

"The wisest men follow their own direction."
– Euripides

After all this cold weather in Ohio (where I was working for the marketing guru) and Massachusetts during April, I felt a burning desire to sweat. Summer was coming, and I wanted to feel some heat although I didn't feel like working out hard enough to really perspire. Good sense told me that I could either pee it out, poop it out, breathe it out or sweat it out. I felt the need to get ALL OF IT out.

The weather was heating up in South Carolina. One day I decided to wear cotton pants, a cotton flannel, and a pair of sweat pants. I also had two hats on. I went outside and made myself jog a few seconds at a time, while walking fast between each jog. I started to sweat just a bit, and then I ran and got into my car, which had been parked in the sun all day. It was well over 130 degrees in the car. I sat in there until I couldn't take it any longer and sweat came through the final layer of clothing. This was my "infrared sauna," and it was awesome! Of course, I brought about 20 oz of water with juice mixed in so that I wouldn't pass out. The point wasn't to make me ill – it was to get me better.

I did this once a week over the entire summer. If I felt like it was too much on my body, I stopped. Once like I felt like I had enough, I stopped. I was getting relief from this self-induced sweat fest! Each time I got out of the car, my flesh looked like a honey baked ham, dripping with sweat as if I had jumped into a swimming pool with all my clothes on.

I had no idea that what I was doing was exactly what doctors do in Europe with a treatment called Hyperthermia. Most people know what hypothermia is (you see it all the time when little Timmies stray from the cub scout group and find themselves wet, cold and alone in the middle of the woods for days). Hyperthermia is the opposite. It's when your internal temperature heats up. Of course in a medical environment, it's controlled. I was going renegade because there is no such hyperthermia treatment in the United States. Hyperthermia is used quite successfully against all types of infection and even cancer in Europe.

My theory for jumping in the car was that I needed to sweat my toxins out, but I was also training my immune system. Back in the old days people got fevers and this was a good thing, it meant your body was fighting back and once the fever broke, you knew everything was going to be okay. I was giving myself a self induced fever, twice a week. I was not only killing Lyme, but probably other types of bacteria and viruses, and training my immune system to fight.

Visiting My Kinesiologist

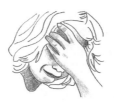

"Desire for security keeps littleness little and
threatens the great with smallness."
– Author Unknown

I kept plugging away for answers about my health. I'd already seen Dr. James, the Lyme disease doctor, and then fired him quickly thereafter. I had been pumping up my immune system with Dr. Rachel, the integrative medical doctor and had just started seeing Dr. Cady. My health was much better overall and I was feeling much more confident, I decided to go to see the world renowned kinesiologist who had helped me diagnose my food allergies at the end of my college years.

He was a young triathlete. It's always great to have doctors who are sports enthusiasts because they seem to understand how important it is for people to keep up with athletics and stay well enough to be able to participate in sports if they choose too. Dr. G works in the university area of North Carolina, so the 4-hour drive there wasn't fun, but I decided to go anyway. My mother went with me as I did not want to drive 8 hours by myself. I brought along my most recent blood work to see if he could use it.

I considered Dr. G a friend, and we have many things in common, including our sense of humor. Applied kinesiology is interesting. It's the study of how people respond to different chemicals, smells, nutrients, etc. Really well-trained doctors can actually tap you, rub you, and muscle test you to get a diagnosis. People are sometimes surprised at how often these diagnoses are the same as what traditional diagnostic testing indicates. But instead of getting expensive blood work, getting stuck with needles, waiting weeks for your results and then having a doctor interpret them, you basically get immediate satisfaction and answers right away.

Dr. G had gotten a lot of business from us in the past. My family referred other people to him, and Dr. G built his practice quite quickly. This time my visit was not so great.

I told Dr. G of my medical problem and gave him my blood work. He did some testing and didn't find any conclusive problems. Perhaps my body was just not being able to be read because it was so incredibly screwed up.

After asking Dr. G what he thought about a particular blood test I had done and how I thought about getting some more, he became angry. He told me that I was making up excuses for not running (of course he didn't phrase it that way, but that's basically what he was getting at). He told me that if I had any more blood work done, he wouldn't see me.

I never saw him again. I was deeply hurt, and cried all the way home in the car. It was devastating to be going to someone for help and have them tell you you're a liar to your face while you are sick.

At some point, when you're on your road to recovery, somebody, whether it's a friend, a family member or your doctor, is going to treat you like a hypochondriac. And when it happens it's hurtful, but you can't expect everyone to understand everything about chronic diseases.

I knew there was something better out there but at this point I wasn't sure what it was. I was just dedicated to figuring it out and trying everything for better or worse. I was going to experiment on myself until I cured myself completely.

One good thing came out of that visit. I left that day with a bottle of NT Factor®, a natural medicine for the fatigue associated with many autoimmune diseases. This was new to me. NT Factor is a formula of phospholipids and glycolipids to be used to repair cellular membranes thus restoring the energy production of cells. See **Appendix XXI** for more information and how to order. Taking it actually helped. I was able to start jogging a bit after taking this.

Back to Exercising

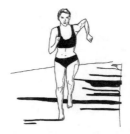

*"Most people never run far enough on their first
wind to find out they've got a second."*
– William James

I was angry at Dr. G, but I took the NT Factor and was getting the IV vitamin C, working on a few deficiency problems with Dr. Rachel and Dr. Cady, and getting back to running. In 2006 I felt like there was hope again. My 10-minute walks had turned into 10-minute runs.

I was still sleeping a lot, about 11 hours a day. (My normal is 9 so I still apparently needed more rest.) In March I was running 25 minutes on good days. The absolute worst was behind me, but there were still many issues that I felt weren't resolved.

I was now able to drive myself to treatment, and I could exercise although not consistently. My body wanted to be better, and I think I had resolved many of the emotional issues that were tied to my health. I had forgiven everyone and didn't do so superciliously. I had carried a lump in my throat (just a constant tightness) from all the anger I had (Dr. Cady brought that to my attention). My lump was gone, even when I recalled stressful situations or trauma that I had witnesses or been a part of during my life. I had "healing reactions," mostly in my armpits above my lymph nodes and in my groin area above my lymph nodes. Sometimes I would also get them on the bottom of my feet (a place where toxins like to gather).

Dr. Rachel gave me another Lyme test in the middle of the year in 2006. It looked almost identical to the one before, except the overall result of the IgM (recurrent or persistent infection) was now negative, not indeterminate (IND). The IgG (recent or chronic infection) was still negative. Did this mean I was doing well? I later had a Russian tick doctor tell me that my results didn't indicate I was doing better or worse.

Looking back, I don't know if it was important to get the Lyme test again. It was important at the beginning to try to obtain the diagnosis. But having that test done didn't make me do anything differently. In fact, because I still didn't feel right, I knew I had to keep going. I was still after answers and knew it wasn't over. Once I realized that the results of the Lyme test weren't going to change my actions, I resolved not to get another one.

Eventually, I felt like I had gotten everything I could from Dr. Rachel and Dr. Cady. I'm glad I saw both of them, but I knew there was something else. I had a meeting with Dr. Rachel, the integrative doctor, and from our discussion, it sounded like she didn't know what more she could do for me.

I was trying hard to believe it was just that and not because she had lost interest.

I had more questions and she didn't have the answers. I wanted to keep figuring things out, and I don't think she believed there was anything else I could do.

She recommended that I see a famous tick doctor up North, but I felt like that was going backwards. One call on her end, referring me up there, would have been better than me calling and finding out that he didn't even see patients anymore. Besides, I had done the traditional Lyme Literate Medical Doctor (LLMD), antibiotic approach. I knew he didn't have the answers I was looking for anyway and "seeing" a doctor who lived far away in another state, somehow didn't make much sense to me.

My time was up with Dr. Rachel. I had gotten what I could from her and then I pressed on, without her.

I still saw Dr. Cady from time to time, but instinctively I knew that I had a brewing problem that was beyond her complete care (soon however, I would find out what it was).

Time for a Break

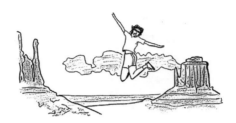

*"The road to success is dotted with many
tempting parking places."*
– Author Unknown

I had been going at this Lyme thing since 2005, and it had been well over a year. I was back to exercising regularly again, and even though I could tell I still had multiple issues left unresolved, I felt good enough to go on a physically active adventure. I wanted to be outside, commune with the great outdoors and live a little. There had been too much sadness, worry and stress over the past months. I decided to take a trip to Arizona and Utah. I just picked places that I thought were interesting and went.

After my trip I was able to exercise even harder, at times even comparable to what I would do on an easy to medium day as an athlete. I could exercise consistently, and while I had better days, I would occasionally regress ever so slightly for a few days or a few weeks. But the interesting thing is this; during this entire ordeal, my highs kept getting higher. But so did my lows! When I regressed (or relapsed), it never was as bad as it was the last time I regressed. The definition of a good day got more exciting as good days were getting WAY BETTER.

I still had a ways to go, but I could see serious progress and that verified that what I was doing was indeed working.

Death of a Friend

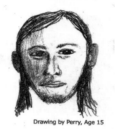

Drawing by Perry, Age 15

"What is death to a caterpillar,
to the butterfly is being set free."
– Author Unknown

I was feeling better and started to feel more optimistic about my recovery. My mother and I were eating lunch one afternoon at this restaurant with a penguin theme. Over lunch we talked about my progress.

I told my mother that since I was feeling better, I wanted to get back in touch with John, one of my best friends. We had met on the first day of art class in high school. I was seated across from him. John had kept all of the art class bullies away by taking them outside after class one day when the bullying had risen to an all time high. I was never bothered again and we became good friends. He even made me a mixed tape. (And, of course, I still have it.)

John was from a broken family with two alcoholic parents,

and to make things worse he was the sensitive-type. He was a deep thinker, all the problems of the world were his problems and he just hated that people did the terrible things they did. Even though he had a problem with drugs and alcohol, we always had a strong bond.

When I told my mother that day at lunch that I wanted to get back in touch, I never could have guessed what was going to come out of her mouth next. All of a sudden, she looked upset and her voice cracked as she said, "Perry, I can't lie to you about this. He's dead….He shot himself about a year ago. I couldn't tell you last year because you were too sick." I felt like my world had just fallen apart…again. I asked a lot of questions, but she had no answers. My sister who had kept in touch with some of her high school friends had been told. She and John were in the same grade.

I had missed his funeral. I had no answers other than he invited friends over to a party of sorts at his mother's house on Lake Murray. Before his friends arrived, he shot himself.

The last time I had seen him we had gotten into an argument while he was intoxicated. I kept replaying that last conversation over and over, wondering what I could have done differently. I had walked out on him that night. I was so hurt by his words. Maybe he was trying to push everyone away so that he could finally do what he had wanted to do for a long time.

It was a shocking reminder that life continues to happen even when you're sick. It was still almost unbearable to deal with even a year later so I went to my parent's house after lunch and went through all of my boxed-up things in the garage looking for every picture I had of him, everything he had ever given me, the yearbooks that had his photo in them, the postcards he had sent me. One of my favorites was a postcard from Venice Beach, CA, that ended with "aren't you glad you have such a good friend like me. Love, John." It was all I had left.

The guilt of not being around when John killed himself and the sadness made me quite ill for weeks afterwards. This was one of the few times when I really regressed even though I was doing all the right things to get my health back. I realized at this time how important emotions are in the healing process, especially trying to get over a serious illness. Being sad can hinder your health, just like stress.

Unfortunately I still have not been able to make peace. The hole in my heart has healed, but it's covered with scar tissue. One day I'll get brave and go to his grave and say good- bye.

My Mountain Doctor

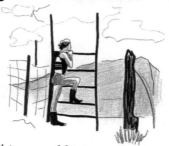

*"The best things and best people rise out of their
separateness. I'm against a homogenized society because
I want the cream to rise to the top."*
– Robert Frost

A fter I got the news about John's death, I had to keep going. John's death made me want to live even more. I wanted to set myself free from this affliction and move on with my life. A friend of my parent's was telling them about his "mountain doctor." As a person with constant health issues, including heart problems, he was having amazing success with his new doc and was telling me about his out-of-the-box thinking. In November of 2006, I went to see this doctor. I didn't expect him to really live like a mountain man. This guy lived up in the most remote section of the Blue Ridge Mountains, in a compound at the end of a service road that stretched for miles to the base of his own private mountain, in a cabin that was built in the 1800's.

I had to go through an interview process just to see this crazy guy. He wasn't even a medical doctor. He got kicked out of South Carolina for practicing without a medical license and his office was raided. I personally don't care what the medical board thinks. I don't think they are always out for my best interest with the things they approve and the things they won't. It looks like a damn conspiracy.

I hate to be a "conspiracy person" because I'm really not. But honestly, what they do doesn't look honorable to me. If I relied on politicians, the government, pharmaceutical companies, and conventional doctors who have to practice in a certain way and abide by all of these rules, I would never have beaten Lyme disease and that's a cold hard fact.

I used my own judgment to see Dr. Bob. My gut feeling has kept me from injury, helped me find a cure for the incurable, and in several situations it has kept me from catastrophic accidents. My gut instinct is what kept pushing me forward during my illness and led me to the mountains to find more answers.

The first day I drove up with my mom, I wondered what had I gotten myself into as I pulled up and this pack of dogs come running out, barking like mad. (We later became BFFs). There was a sign on a post that said "Trespassing fine $50,000."

I was kind of worried at this point. I saw chickens running around everywhere, some sheep, some cats, a pack of dogs and nobody in sight. This wasn't your usual health care facility, but come to find out, I'd be spending a whole lot of time up there.

So this guy, Dr. Bob, who looked like a Civil War veteran,

came out and we went into this pre-Civil War cabin – his office.

We talked and he gave me more information than I knew what to do with about why people become diseased, the breakdown of our current medical system and even problems with agriculture and the impact of nutritional deficiencies on our society. Dr. Bob, had conducted cancer research and told me what he thought the cure actually was. I believe he may be right, because the closest cure for Lyme was actually the same as his theoretical cancer cure.

He was so earnest that my mother decided to get a work up while she was there as well.

He had his assistant put some straps around our ankles, wrists and head and used a bio feedback machine to do his work up. Imagine technology like this sitting inside a pre-Civil War cabin. It felt like I was on a prank show and I was getting Punk'd.

Thermal Imaging

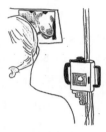

*"You can judge your age by the amount of pain you
feel when you come in contact with a new idea."*
– Author Unknown

The first thing I got was a thermal image of my entire body. Thermal imaging (referred to as thermography) is really fascinating. It uses a highly specialized infrared camera that can measure thermal patterns. Thermal patterns can be an indication of where inflammation and disease are and directly correlates to pain, injury or some other type of abnormality. They can even detect tiny little spots in the breasts that are precancerous (ones that mammograms can't even detect). The best thing about it is that you don't have to touch anything. You aren't poked and prodded. You just strip down, stand in front of this camera, and it takes pictures. Yes, you might have to get over the shyness for this one, but it's worth it.

My test results weren't ready that day, so I didn't get to see where the inflammation was. The test results were interpreted by another medical group (see the results in **Appendix X** to get an idea of what you can expect).

I had a number of serious issues that came up, but the test results went on to describe other areas that were totally fine. My breast area was fine, no findings of anything cancerous or any inflammation being there. Finally, good news...my breasts were going to be okay! Not that I was worried about my boobs, but at that point I felt like I was a potential candidate for EVERYTHING. I have to admit I thought the testing was pretty accurate, knowing what I had been experiencing. The back reading was dead on because my back, right below the site of my bite, had been itchy and tingly for quite some time. I knew it was inflamed, but this was the proof. I had an enormous angry red and yellow pattern stemming from the exact location of my tick bite behind my neck, going half way down my back.

The most important feedback from the test was that Dr. Bob said we needed a closer look in my mouth because he was sure something was not right. The official reading did not indicate that I had anything wrong with my mouth, probably because the thermal image only showed very weak color changes in my mouth, but Dr. Bob was sure I had pathology in my mouth.

Bioscience: Blood Analysis

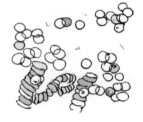

"A lot of good arguments are spoiled by some fool
who knows what he is talking about."
– Author Unknown

D r. Bob also used darkfield microscopy to analyze my blood. He looked at a wet sample and a dry sample, to formulate an opinion about what was going on inside. To perform this analysis a dab of blood is placed on a glass slide and the blood cells are viewed under a special microscope.

This is a way of looking at the biological issues affecting health. With this type of screening, factors such as oxidation, cholesterol, fibrinogen levels, build up of calcium deposits and plaque are all checked (to see my complete results and Dr. Bob's explanation, see **Appendix XI**). A high powered microscope is used to evaluate blood cells and while this method is not considered a diagnostic procedure, it is pretty good at evaluating different conditions that one's blood is describing.

The most notable problems that Dr. Bob saw were "ghost cells" (when a blood cell has lost its hemoglobin and the membrane is the only thing observed), which indicated anemia. It meant I was iron deficient. (Hemolysis is what people with anemia have, where the busted blood cell releases hemoglobin into the surrounding plasma.) What perplexed me about this was that I had had a hemoglobin test with Dr. Rachel, the integrative medical doctor, but she hadn't tested me for ferritin. Ferritin is the storage of iron in the body, and a low score here is the best indication that you're crashing from low iron or you have already crashed.

Back at Clemson in 2002, I became terribly iron deficient during the end of my outdoor track season. I forced the team doctor to give me a blood work up. My ferritin was a 3. Now everyone's natural levels are different, but a 3 pretty much indicates a very big anemic problem, no matter who you are. A normal level for someone like me might be 40, and for someone else it might be 80. Men typically have higher levels than women. Getting routine testing will let you know when you have a problem. The easiest way is just to get a wet sample of your blood looked at under a microscope.

Dr. Bob then looked at a dried blood sample. Bingo! I had one of the worst cases of parasites he'd ever seen. Using darkfield microscopy it isn't easy or even feasible in some cases to identity the various types. Most of these parasites came from years of living like most people, from food, water, traveling, pets, even walking on soil with bare feet, it clearly adds up over time. He then told me of one case worse than mine. It was a girl who worked in a mortuary embalming dead bodies. She had to go to the ER when she started to rid herself of parasites because of the toxin overload caused from the die-off.

As he looked deeper at my blood work he discovered that I also had a very high score for heavy metals.

I left that first day with some insight into what exactly was plaguing me. I was told to have my oral pathology corrected, remove my parasites using a parasite kit, take these fermented soybean enzymes, take a diabetic pack (to clean my receptor sites since I was becoming partially diabetic), take a nano form of iron, keep taking iodine and come see him again.

Taking Enzymes and Fixing Anemia

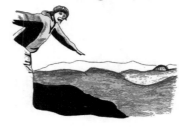

"When the world says, 'Give up,'
Hope whispers, "Try it one more time."
– Author Unknown

I started taking the enzymes that were developed somewhere nearby in South Carolina by fermenting soybeans. Dr. Bob mixed a micronized iron formula into the enzyme juice. On my next visit the ghost cells were gone, and this was within 30 days! I thought this was near impossible because when you crash with anemia it usually takes months to build up your ferritin storage (as it did my senior year at Clemson University). I always had Coach, from Tucson, telling me to watch out for this as he coached many professional athletes who bombed out due to anemic conditions and took anywhere from a couple of months to a full year to recover (sometimes longer). I was feeling so much better on the enzymes just because I wasn't totally exhausted anymore.

The enzymes were interesting because I was speaking with other patients of Dr. Bob, many of whom had clogged arteries and a fibrinogen mess in their bodies. After taking this enzyme, many of them would return to their regular doctors for routine testing. Their doctors were flabbergasted by arteries mysteriously becoming unclogged and fibrinogen levels and calcium deposits going down dramatically. They would say, "My mountain doctor gave me these enzymes," and their regular doctors would say, "Well, keep taking them!"

I felt like I was drinking some type of bootleg mixture (from *way up yonder in the mountains*). It was just fermented soybeans, using some special process. (See **Appendix XII** about the enzymes).

Natto is another form of fermented soybeans that looks like a white powder. In the future two other doctors also gave me Nattokinase (NK), which is a fibrinolytic enzyme of natto. This enzyme dissolves blood clots and prevents heart attacks when clotting gets stuck in high gear. This enzyme reverses blood clotting, and regulates it, modulating the process by re-establishing coagulation homeostasis.

Natto has been a traditional Japanese staple for over 1,000 years. Its medical benefits have been widely recognized. It is purported to prevent heart attacks, strokes, cancer, osteoporosis, intestinal disease caused by pathogens and obesity. As the bacteria natto (bacillus natto) ferments, it produces enzymes, vitamins, amino acids and other nutrients that are essential to good health.

So, in essence, this was a "fix it all" enzyme. I always heard other patients talk so highly of these enzymes. In fact some of these former heart attack victims left the care of their cardiologist because they were "miraculously" healed and their levels of fibrinogen dropped off so sharply that their own "real" doctors were amazed.

As with most diseases, Lyme had left me with many deficiencies and the enzymes seemed to be filling many needs. The inflammation found in the thermal image was more than likely due to excessive fibrinogen levels in me as well. I recently read about various health conditions due to excessive fibrinogen levels. Here are just a few: angina, thrombosis, stroke, heart disease, chronic fatigue, fibromyalgia, varicose veins, muscle spasm, poor healing, chronic inflammation and pain, hypertension, infertility, tissue oxygen deprivation and gynecologic conditions, just to name a few. You can get more information on these metabolic enzymes by visiting: *www.TheTickSlayer.com/enzymes.*

Fixing Blood Sugar Problems

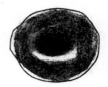

"I am on the verge of mysteries and the veil is getting thinner and thinner."
– Louis Pasteur

I never thought I had diabetes, but I took this product for blood sugar support (see **Appendix XIII** for more information). I did have a problem with blood sugar, so I guess maybe diabetes was on the way.

When I was little I would go wild if I had just a tiny taste of sugar, becoming completely unable to control myself, sometimes laughing and crying at the same time. It was like a drug. I remember being little and having a sugar high in the back of the car beside my sister on a family trip. These usually resulted in spankings (with hands on the trunk of the car so that everyone driving past could see). I wasn't bad, I just couldn't control myself. I suspect a lot of young kids today are this way. As I got older, this settled down a bit, but if I did not eat at regular intervals, I would have slumps that I thought would kill me. So obviously something was imbalanced.

The blood sugar support pack reduced blood sugar levels and helped control the cause of diabetes by cleaning the receptor sites that process sugar in the body. These receptor sites help the body balance proper glucose levels. When these sites become overloaded, your body wigs out when it gets sugar or a food that converts to glucose quickly (like white bread, pasta, and refined foods). Some symptoms of a blood sugar problem are poor energy, weight issues, sleeping problems, constant thirst or frequent urination, pain and tingling in the feet or hands and dry skin.

The product I took contained various supplements that needed to be taken at certain times of the day. These supplements included chromium, magnesium, molybdenum and vanadium, essential fatty acids (EFAs) and corosolic acid (which has been shown to enhance glucose transport without any side effects). I personally didn't notice a huge change, but perhaps my biggest blood sugar issues were behind me at this point. Taking them had no adverse effects and only strengthened my overall well-being. Eating a gluten-free diet and naturally avoiding processed or refined foods may control this issue naturally, since most gluten containing foods spike insulin quickly.

Oral Pathology is Killing Everyone

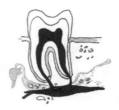

"It is easier to believe a lie that one has heard
a thousand times than to believe a fact that no
one has heard before."
– Author Unknown

I had my wisdom teeth removed in 1999, my sophomore year in college. My jaw was just too tiny and they were crowding my front teeth, which had already been straightened by braces (for cosmetic, but mostly mechanical reasons as I couldn't bite a spaghetti quill in half). I went to a well respected dental surgeon in South Carolina to have them removed. This dentist had done thousands of surgeries like this, and it is still a pretty common surgery for kids that age to have.

I never had any other serious dental problems. I have only had two cavities to this very day! Both are filled with nontoxic, plastic "composite" fillings.

I found out that many people who have had major dental

work done like wisdom teeth removal, metal fillings, root canals, bridges or pins have an elevated risk of being ill, without any knowledge of the source of the illness. The scary part is you may not even have pain your mouth to indicate a problem. I certainly never felt any pain.

On Dr. Bob's recommendation I went to see these two biological dentists in Tennessee, who go about dentistry in a holistic way, specifically look for toxicity or dysfunction in the teeth and jaws. There aren't many in the U.S. because they are scrutinized by the American Dental Association which thinks its traditional dentists aren't doing anything wrong. These biological dentists don't like to make a big stink about what they are doing for fear of losing their licenses. The truth is oral pathology due to a previous surgery is a VERY big deal and it has to be cleaned up so that an individual can regain their health completely from major illness. This is a very sad issue and it's appalling to me that I had to go to such great lengths to even be aware of this issue. Had I not found out about this, I might not have ever gotten over Lyme disease completely.

If you have disease in your mouth, your body's immune system stays suppressed, and overtime you become increasingly susceptible to illnesses like Lyme, cancer and other autoimmune diseases. Most diseases, if not all, are diseases of opportunity. Infections can fester in areas where your body is weak.

I was curious to see what these dentists would say. I had Dr. Bob look at my mouth right before I left with a Cavitat™, a machine that detects necrosis in the jawbone by projecting a 3-D color image of the infected area using ultrasound. It picks up on the diseased area, and you get results right then and there. The machine is FDA cleared, but its use has been met with resistance from mainstream groups like the American Dental Association (ADA) and various insurance companies. When there is a difference of opinion, you are going to have a lot of people pointing fingers at each other. I could see why the American Dental Association thumbs their nose at this, root canals are profitable business and insurance companies… well, they don't want to pay for anything. Just take a look at how much the CEOs of insurance companies make (it's in the hundreds of millions to the billion dollar range). I don't think it's criminal to make a ton of money, but making ridiculous amounts of money by denying people coverage of important health care treatment is a 1,000% percent wrong. Yet another reason why it's important to follow your own instincts.

The Cavitat gets its name from "cavitations," which are lesions that can produce toxins, and are often located in old extraction sites or near the roots of root canal teeth, dead teeth and wisdom teeth. Sometimes these cavitations spread from these locations throughout the jawbone and penetrate the sinus cavity. If these cavitations are not cleaned, they can cause jaw necrosis (diseased jaw bone).

These lesions are neurotoxic and not only contribute to cancer but also keep people with Lyme disease, and other serious diseases from becoming disease-free. I believe that people who have difficulty recovering from any type of autoimmune disease may have jaw necrosis. Dr. Bob said he's researched thousands of cases, and every time someone comes to him with cancer, they also have jaw necrosis, on the same side of the body as the cancer. Investigative data show an incredibly high percentage of old extraction sites from wisdom teeth removal and all teeth treated with root canal therapy have cavitational lesions[1].

The worst part may be the fact that insurance companies consider the surgery to clean up these cavitation sites to be "elective" surgery, which puts it in the same category as plastic surgery! But if the dentist takes a sample of the infected jaw bone and has it tested for being necrotic (as in "rotted"), it now becomes surgery you need and insurance may cover it.

So this entire time that I felt like something was still wrong, I was right! Gut feeling wins again. I knew something was suppressing my immune system. I knew there was a bigger issue, and this was it! Because of my experience, I don't have to die of cancer or from Lyme disease in ten or twenty years, and neither does my family. Maybe I can help save the lives of thousands of other people who read this book. I made my mother, father and sister get their "dental cleanup" done, and my sister was on the way to getting cancer as she had a lump in her breast that correlated to the oral pathology in her mouth -on the same side of her body (just like Dr. Bob said).

During the dental visit, this dentist in Tennessee took an x-ray and pointed out little specks that no other dentist would even notice. He said he suspected that I had problems under three of the four wisdom teeth extraction sites. The surgery for this was interesting. The dentist in Tennessee didn't use the Cavitat, nor did they use any other method for detection, and later on I was pissed off that they hadn't, as my sites were re-infected later on because they were not fully cleaned

1. Wesley Shankland, "NICO And Cavitations," The Doctor's Medical Library, http://www.medical-library.net/content/view/135/41/ (accessed October 28, 2011).

out. I found out later it takes a very aggressive surgeon to remove all of this mess, the use of the Cavitat and an electro-acupuncture testing device should be used to make sure all of the toxic material is removed.

During surgery, I was nervous but I ponied up like a real cowgirl. I had just finished another salt and C protocol for Lyme, and the vitamin C was apparently detoxing the Novocain too fast. I had so many injections that the dentist gave me epinephrine. Now, as I said earlier because of my genomic test, I knew that I don't detox this stuff well, but I forgot to mention that to the dentist. I was at my legal limit of Novocain with one more injection, because of my body weight, I could only have so much in one sitting. When the dentist gave me the epinephrine, my body went into shock. The color drained from my face, and I started bucking like a wild horse, trying to keep myself from passing out. The dentist put ice packs in my crotch and armpits. After what seemed like an hour, I was almost normal again, and by this time I was super numb in the mouth.

Once the dentist started drilling into the jawbone, they tapped into the cavitation holding all of this toxicity and this 'black oil' slipped down my throat. They caught most of it with a little vacuuming instrument, but the taste was enough to make me want to vomit. Oddly enough, I felt a huge surge of energy, like a huge weight was lifted off my shoulders and out of my body. The dentist tapped the other two sites and did a little scraping.

Later, I found out he needed to do more than just drain it. He needed to physically scrape the infection out to remove all of it. What hurt me most is that later on I found out they knew about the Cavitat and other technology, but just weren't incorporating it into their practice. Had they used it, they could have tested right then and there to make sure the diseased part was removed completely. I was thinking this problem was solved, but later on I would have to revisit it again.

By late December 2006, I had finished my dental surgery to get rid of the infection in my jaw. This was one short month after my initial visit to Dr. Bob, who said to go get my oral pathology fixed. I wasn't letting grass grow under my feet!

I was feeling better than ever before. I felt like I was on track, and I could see the finish line. I even started to do hard workouts just to test myself, but I still felt like something was off, so I kept going, looking for more answers.

Energetic Medicine Kicks Ass

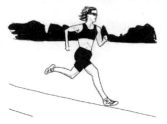

"Science does not know its debt to imagination."
– Ralph Waldo Emerson

Energetic medicine is the term used to describe how quantum physics is being used as medicine to treat people with various ailments. Acupuncture, reiki, aromatherapy are all forms of energetic medicine. However, the technology (by way of manufactured devices) harnessing frequency and vibrations to counter specific conditions is rapidly growing, although it's not fully embarrassed by western medicine.

Almost every weekend I drove up to the mountains to teach myself how to use Dr. Bob's energetic medicine machines. While using them, I started to take notes on how these things work, how they made me feel (from a research perspective). I was experimenting on myself to see what worked and what didn't because my desire to understand things is like curiosity in cats. It can't always be controlled.

Dr. Bob was very scattered-brained. I knew he was smart, but I only had one phone number to reach him at (the number to the phone in the pre-Civil War cabin that was his "clinic" of sorts). So if no one was in the cabin, which was usually the case, I had to drive up 3 hrs to talk to him. Sometimes as I would leave after an appointment with him we would agree on a time for me to come again (usually the next weekend so I could work on the machines when no one else would need them). I always wanted to call before I came up, but sometimes I just had to drive up and hope that someone would be there to let me in. On some visits I would be locked out of the cabin and have to wait with the free range chickens on the front porch. (We had an agreement, if they didn't poop on me, I wouldn't chase them around.) Then, Dr. Bob would come walking out of nowhere, talking about how he had to fix this or that fence, or move these rocks or feed this animal or clear that brush, etc. etc.

Dr. Bob knew I was smart enough to teach myself how to use the machines, and he took an interest in me. I was a special project of sorts. Because it took 3 hrs to drive there (in winter, on icy, slick mountain roads) I usually stayed at least one night before heading home. Unfortunately, this place was in the coldest part of the Blue Ridge Mountains. It was at an elevation of about 5,000 feet and it was in a bit of a valley so no direct sunlight ever hit the cabin except at high noon, then the sun would dip behind the mountains as fast as it had risen above them. The cabin had one little heater connected to the wall in the "office." The sofa that turned into the bed was the closest sleeping area to that heater. So, that is where I slept.

During January, I spent all day in my mountain parka (having a down-filled coat was essential) because it was so cold (sometimes staying in the 20's) during the day. At night it dropped into the negatives. The sheep would huddle together, the chickens got quiet (and went somewhere), the cats disappeared and the Great Pyrenees dogs just slept against the cabin door like it was summertime. On those nights I used every wool blanket in the cabin and slept in all of my clothes and my down parka in my sleeping bag rated below freezing, and I would still wake up with chill on my face. I was happy when the chickens and roosters let me know at the crack of dawn that morning was indeed coming.

Sometimes I got up and fed the farm animals simply because I couldn't get anything done until I had fed them. The cabin sat flush against the fence of their meadow, and everyone gathered in the morning making all kinds of noises until they were fed. I sure did step in a lot of shit those mornings--that's why the boots came off before going back inside!

Over time, the guard dogs became my buddies, and between treatments I would take them for walks through the mountains, which they loved. One would run behind me, one beside me and one ahead of me (the male dog, of course).

I never walked around in the woods or up to the top of the mountain without the dogs as Dr. Bob warned me about a cougar that was eating his animals. I believe I heard it one night because the chickens were stirring. I felt sorry for the cougar also because Dr. Bob's property was sitting beside some of the last mountain tops that were completely uninhabited by people. The farm animals were just easy meals, and the mother cougar had babies to feed.

I loved walking around with the dogs up and around the mountains. This area of the mountains had incredibly pure spring water all over. I felt like I had a little piece of heaven. I spent a lot of time thinking about what I was doing and how I was going to get over this. I was daydreaming of racing again. Walking up hills turned into running up hills, and every time I went for treatment with these machines I felt better and better. I started to bring my running clothes, and I began to exercise more and more.

It obviously wasn't the type of "healthcare" most people think of, but it sure beats the hell out of sitting in the traditional dismal waiting room surrounded by sickness. If that isn't doom and gloom I don't know what is. This felt right to me even though driving up the first day and seeing this "compound" of sorts, startled me.

QXCI

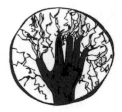

"Don't have a battle of wits with an unarmed opponent."
– Anonymous

I got hooked up to a QXCI (which is a type of energetic medicine machine) to test my cellular values during my first visit with Dr. Bob. All cells have voltage, amperage, resistance, hydration and oxygen values. Voltage reflects adrenal values; amperage shows brain function serotonin; resistance reflects ease of flow of energy through the body; hydration reveals ease of water; and oxygen shows the flow of oxygen and oxygenation through the body. My scores were pretty bad on these, but with a little therapy on this machine, which I'll explain in detail later, my scores started to improve.

People using Rife machines (machines that use frequencies to kill bacteria and other pathogens) will be more inclined to understand the benefits of using energetic medicine. I'm compelled to tell you about the device because in my journey, I experimented with a lot of unconventional treatments and it's why I had success. I just put myself out there. When conventional medicine fails to treat diseases people become more open to alternative care, and rightfully so. The science behind energetic medicine is very real, although opponents of this particular device believe it's phony. Some of it is based on theories (and that's the argument against it), but what's amazing is that electricity is just a theory also; nobody really knows exactly how it happens. Science is so cool.

It's hard for most people to comprehend but everything in the universe is a sea of floating molecules end-on-end. Every molecule of matter, depending on its structure, resonates at a different frequency and even emotions have vibrations. Every cell has an intelligent energetic pattern that the QXCI supposedly detects. Diseases, organs, pathogens, nutrients, allergens, even emotions all have different energetic frequencies that they transmit. The QXCI can audit a person's physical, emotional, mental and spiritual health. Emotions cause strong physical reactions; therefore, they can be tested. In a just few minutes about 8,000 measurements can be obtained with this machine.

I was seriously intrigued by the QXCI, as it was my first encounter with anything in the energetic medicine realm. It had head, wrist and ankle straps and can apparently work over long distances without the straps, much like someone praying for you from afar. This falls inside the realm of radionics. I have a good understanding of space, matter, the universe, the world, particle matter and how science can explain a lot of it, but there are some parts that will always be a mystery.

The QXCI can be helpful in telling you what your deficiencies are, what works well and what needs improvement, what diseases you have or have been exposed too (those are two different things) and what organ systems are stressed. It also gives you suggestions on what you can do and what you can take to rebuild your health. The strangest part is that for every issue you might have, there is a frequency the machine can send to help you balance yourself.

The enormous downfall to the machine is that you constantly wonder how accurate the results are. It can drive you insane knowing about all the issues keeping you constantly unbalanced. Every day your body chemistry changes due to internal and external factors. This is life. Our bodies are constantly trying to stay balanced, so it makes senses for values to change so suddenly.

As I played around with the machine, I realized that it could detect emotions and that I could use it to give myself therapy for different stressors. I would test my emotions, and my number one issue that always came up was RESENTMENT. Now, after reading a little about my athletic life, can you see maybe why this would keep coming up? So I actually worked on this for months, not only "zapping" my resentment but doing techniques to just let things go. That night, two years ago, when I was so sick, screaming and lying naked on the floor with my body going crazy, I let a lot of things go because I thought I was going to die. Now it seemed like I had more personal issues I had to work on. This damn machine would always tell me "less judgment and more acceptance." I got the point QXCI, thank you.

My mom would come with me on the weekends, and I

started using the machine on her. I got so tickled because I tested her emotions to see what she wasn't telling me! She had no idea what I was testing, and then I would say, "So, mom, I see that you are suppressing your anger; would you like to talk about it?" My mom is the type of person who always seems cheery even though she might be burning with anger on the inside. She doesn't want anyone to say anything bad to anyone else, so she keeps things inside, just simmering away. The QXCI couldn't have been more right about it. So once I finally got my mother to admit that she did feel anger, I worked on her emotions as well.

There was basic testing you could do to find out issues, at first my list was long, but after a few months, it was pretty well cleaned up. If that machine gave me a suggestion for what to take, I would take it. If it told me emotional things I should work on, I did. Probably the hardest thing to decipher was what it told me about cancer: I may not have cancer, but if I was around someone who did, the frequency from the cancer could very well show up on my QXCI reading. This happened several times with my mother and myself. A client who had cancer came into my parent's office right before my mother and I left to go to North Carolina to use the machines. When we started doing our reading, we got a positive reading for cancer. This scared us but, Dr. Bob said these things happen. It didn't mean I had it. The QXCI was just reading frequencies. I might have someone else's frequency on me, but it didn't mean I was sick with it.

When doing a general reading I was assigned a score for various problems. Even health problems that were just a small threat showed up in the results. My readings were dead on for the conditions that I knew I already had, but modern medicine has a hard time testing for conditions that are still "in the works."

The QXCI told me I was iodine deficient (yep, that was true), had irregular menstruation (yep, my entire life), had hypoadrenia (yep, I had already been tested for a adrenal fatigue), had short-term toxicity (yep, that was true, and I had been trying hard to detox), had a malabsorption issue and toxic bowel (yep, I already knew this because of the Gluten issue, and later, I found out from another doctor that I did indeed have permeability issues), had an allergy to wheat and citrus and the QXCI mentioned a few other foods to stay away from (yep, I also have the conventional testing that says this is true), had problems with my dental health (yep, I had already had surgery, but at this time still had no idea the dentist didn't get everything), had parasites (yep, I needed to fix that issue), had a thyroid that needed to be detoxed (yep, I have no idea what that means, but I did have thyroid issue so it makes sense) and told me "forgiveness of God was important." (This never showed up on my mom's, but yep, I was very angry at God and everything else while ill.)

What's interesting is that everything it mentioned was correct, and I either already had the testing to prove it or had testing later (like the problem with my dental health and later finding out I had permeability issues).

So you want to know about the Lyme part right? Yep, the QXCI found it. I was positive for "Lyme Brucellosis"; Brucellosis, Babesia and Rocky Mountain spotted fever. The funniest part was that beside every one, was its definition, and part of the explanation included biological warfare. But,

I'm not going to get into that part. There are other books that explain the U.S. bio warfare lab off the coast of New York. I don't know enough about it. I skimmed those books and decided it was best to remain ignorant (obviously I'm not ignorant about it, but I can't get angry about it. I'm not fighting that battle).

Furthermore, The QXCI can detect little genetic issues and then tell you about them, but you won't know what to do about them (if anything). Frustrating? Not really. I appreciated how aware I was becoming (the term is "biofeedback"); however, the verdict is out as far as the frequencies it can send back to a person to help correct certain issues. The QXCI can send frequencies back to you for healing, but I don't know for sure if 'zapping' yourself with the B12 frequency is as good as taking it. I believe something is better than nothing, and I think my zapping was helpful in balancing myself a little more.

I used the machine about twice a month for 4-5 months. It was instrumental in helping me cope with the emotional side of my illness because it was dead on about the resentment I was still carrying (even though it took a machine to point it out for me to finally deal with it). And I did have a problem with God. I was pissed. Pissed at the world and whoever made Lyme, pissed that I had to be bitten that day, pissed that it took years off my career and almost took my life.

I did the, "Why me, God?" thing once and I never did it again. When this machine told me to forgive, I realized it was totally right. I had to take part, if not most, of the blame. I chose my career path, chose to ignore my feelings, and chose to live the way I was living. I bet there are people out there with the same disease who have never succumbed to it because their lifestyle is so much easier and happier. For me this disease was a real turning point and for that I am grateful.

ONDAMED®

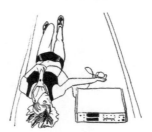

"Nothing has such power to broaden the mind as the
ability to investigate systematically and truly all
that comes under thy observation in life."
– Marcus Aurelius

D
r. Bob had another machine called the ONDAMED. It's more like the "Rife" machines people talk about today (for information on Rife and the ONDAMED see **Appendix XIV**), but much more specific. It uses electromagnetic fields to strengthen the immune system to help combat Lyme, but also acts as a biofeedback machine to pinpoint specific health issues and organs that are distressed or diseased. The ONDAMED is not a radionics device, you have to be present for it to work.

To be clear, you have to understand there are all types of technology out there and new technology is constantly being created. The ONDAMED uses frequencies with electromagnetic fields to pinpoint specific issues.

The old school medical way is based on the chemical model, so medical doctors are taught how to manipulate our bodies using this model. They aren't taught physics. Our bodies are based on electro-magnetism, and the heart is electric. So we can use different models, in addition to the chemical model to help us heal.

For example, our bodies need electrolytes so that our heart keeps ticking, which it does by way of electric current. Do you remember the grade school science experiment where the electricity to run a light bulb comes from an electrolyte solution and metal? It demonstrates how electrolytes can conduct electricity. The heart is like the light bulb, without a conductive fluid it cannot operate.

The ONDAMED uses sound and magnetic pulses to stimulate the body at various frequencies. These identified pulses and frequencies provide feedback as they are measured values applied to certain areas (types of illnesses, emotions, etc.) The ONDAMED can stimulate cell repair and can send frequencies that penetrate the blood-brain barrier. This kind of treatment could be very important to very ill people who have serious neurotransmitter problems associated with disease, stress, diet, etc. Nutrients can cross the blood brain barrier, but so can frequency. Other tick born bacteria (as in other infections that are commonly found in people who have Lyme disease) can often go into the brain and I believe using frequency is one of the best ways to destroy the bacteria without taking the drugs that are commonly prescribed for this (and which often fail in getting all of the infection). For more information on ONDAMED and its uses, see **Appendix 2-II** for details from Rolf Binder and Dr. Silvia Binder.

Multi-Wave Oscillating Machine

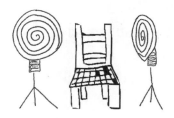

*"You cannot discover new oceans unless you have
the courage to lose sight of the shore."*
– Anonymous

I call the Multi-Wave Oscillator (MWO, for short) the "Pie Tin" machine because it looks like two pie tins on tripod stands. This machine was developed by a French scientist, Georges Lakhovsky in 1920 by using a Tesla coil[1]. Everyone should know who Tesla is, a brilliant scientist, famous for his showdown with Thomas Edison over the AC vs. DC currents. Lakhovsky was a big fan of Tesla's.

Lakhovsky's little machine demonstrated how living cells have a DNA strand that acts like a self- inducting coil. Each cell resonates to external sources of frequencies. According to Lakhovsky, exposing yourself to healthy frequencies induces a detoxification effect.

---

1. Lakhovsky, Georges. 1931. Apparatus with circuits oscillating under multiple wave lengths. US Patent 574,907, filed November 13, 1931, and issued June 12, 1934.

Nikola Tesla said that radiant energy was therapeutic and rejuvenating. Lakhovsky believed in the same idea. He believed living cells were like batteries and could be recharged like a battery if exposed to electromagnetic oscillations. It's a fact that the electrical potentials of a healthy cell and one that is cancerous are quite different because the sodium and potassium are not balanced in cancerous cells. I already knew of the amazing health effects of balancing electrolytes properly, but at this time I had no idea how to do it. This machine "encourages" cells to vibrate in the correct order, allowing important information to be transmitted across cells (allowing cells to communicate, as it were).

When the QXCI tested my cell values, it tested my cell voltage, which was quite poor initially, but using the OXCI and the Multi-Wave Oscillator for only a few treatments, it climbed into the normal range (without taking an electrolyte replacement solution).

Lakhovsky thought that if outside sources of frequencies (like the Multi Wave-Oscillator) were in "sympathy" with the cell, i.e. both producing the same frequency, the cell itself became stronger and healthier. His view of disease was that if the vibrations of cells in the body were not as strong as the vibrations of the virus or bacteria, then the pathogens would win the battle by weakening the rest of the healthy cells energetically, making them more susceptible to disease. Lakhovsky theorized that, "The amplitude of cell oscillations must reach a certain value, in order that the organism be strong enough to repulse the destructive vibrations from certain microbes[2]." What an awesome postulation, I say!

2. Georges Lakhovsky, "Radtiations and Waves, Theory of Cellular Oscillation," Source of Our Life, 1941. http://users.skynet.be/Lakhovsky/Georges_Lakhovsky-Radiation_And_Waves_Sources_Of_Our_Life_1941_OCR.pdf (accessed October 23, 2011)

Lakhovsky conducted experiments on plants, inoculating them with cancer and exposing them to x-rays so that they developed tumors all over. He then used radio frequencies (the same principle behind the Multi-Wave Oscillator) to dry them up. Within a short amount of time and with few treatments, the plants shed the tumors and became vibrant; even the tumors surrounded by healthy cells died, leaving the healthy cells in perfect condition. This science is used today to "blast" cancer tumors in the body.

I used a Multi-Wave Oscillator at Dr. Bob's. I put these pie tins on either side of my head, very close (exposing myself to an enormous number of harmonic frequencies at different wavelengths) and sat in this terribly uncomfortable ancient wooden chair (it worked because the chair kept me sitting up right). These two "tins" were moved around, but always faced each other, and were placed on opposite sides of my body. The closer they got, the more concentrated the frequencies were to that specific area. At first the machine scared me because of the snapping and crackling from the electrical discharge, but not all of these energetic medicine machines make so much noise.

I directed the machine toward my head because I knew that Lyme could live in the brain, causing insanity. Since I had already gone through some serious psychosis, I thought I would just try to get all of it out! I was allowed to do only two sessions (or one hour total) per visit because of the intensity. I never felt bad from doing it. In fact, I never felt bad from doing any of these "experimental" treatments. I only improved. This made me believe that you can really heal many conditions without causing harm, unlike many traditional methods. If we had more healthcare freedom, many doctors would probably embrace the technology that's out there because I believe that many of them do have the intentions to heal their patients with everything that's available.

To get more information on the MWO, see *www.TheTickSlayer.com/MWO*

The Science is Out There

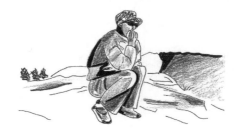

"Anarchy - it's not the law, it's just a good idea."
– Author Unknown

If the machines sound far-fetched, it's understandable. Some devices out there are based far more on measurable efficacy statistics then others. I was watching a program on space when a scientist said the mind is incapable of dealing with the fact that space is infinite. For many people, it's also incapable of understanding how many of the fancy gadgets we use every day (like cell phones) work, never mind that some technology is just 'theory' in action. Our minds are trapped in what happened 5,000 or 10,000 years ago and can't quite get the BIG picture. Then there are some people who can't think of anything but the future. I like to stay somewhere in the middle. A good knowledge of history, excited about the future, but happy and focused on living in the present moment.

Death of My Granny: The Alzheimer's-Lyme Connection

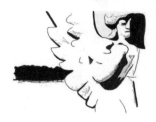

"In the darkest hour the soul is replenished and given strength to continue to endure."
– Heart Warrior Chosa

Even though I had much to be thankful for with finding my way through the Lyme maze and healing myself, life was still going on. Christmas was coming, and I was finishing my last treatments at Dr. Bob's for the year. It was getting harder and harder to drive up to see him because of the weather. The twisting mountain roads with sharp drop-offs were usually covered with ice in the morning and evening. It was time to give it a rest for the holidays.

Christmas that year was going to be at my aunt's house in Columbia, South Carolina, the one and only eccentric sister of my father. She's so active that she could be construed as "overly hyper." My step-uncle has a bait farm, which is strange because it's a nice place, but a few roads down from the ghetto, at the end of the main drag, called Two Notch Road, which was full of hookers and seedy strip clubs at night.

My grandmother got a free Christmas Day pass out of "granny lock down" in the Dementia/Alzheimer's ward on the lower level of a new nursing home near my aunt. My granny had already been kicked out of the first nursing home she was in. She's a bit of a spitfire and apparently slapped some elderly gentleman. She went into a nursing home long before she became physically disabled, because she was a bit mentally disabled (although my dad says she was always crazy). When we were younger, she would tell use to gather for a photo and right before she took the picture, she'd say, "Say Sex!"

It's known that there is a correlation between spirochete bacteria (Lyme bacteria is spirochete in shape) in the brain and dementia and Alzheimer's. St. Catherine of Siena Medical Center Pathologist Dr. Alan B. MacDonald has a hypothesis that a spirochete infection (syphilis), which shows many parallels with Borrelia infections such as Lyme disease, could be the culprit to many brain-wasting diseases like Lou Gehrig's Disease (ALS), Dementia, and Alzheimer's[1]. I wonder how many cases of Alzheimer's disease could be prevented if people knew about the correlation with Lyme disease.

Granny watched the fireworks after supper. We're pretty "red necky" and like to shoot fireworks and yell during Christmas. She was cold so she sat in the car, and looked

1. MacDonald, "Plaques of Alzheimer's disease originate from cysts of Borrelia burgdorferi, the Lyme disease spirochete," MacDonald, "Alzheimer's neuroborreliosis with trans-synaptic spread of infection and neurofibrillary tangles derived from intraneuronal spirochetes,"Visit www.molecularalzheimer.org for information on Dr. MacDonald's studies.

like she wanted to go to sleep. I tapped on the window and told her goodbye and kissed her. That was the last time I saw her, but I knew it would be, I could feel it. A few days after Christmas, she died. I think she was waiting to see everyone one last time.

Oh My God
I'm Full of Parasites

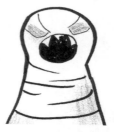

"An effective way to deal with predators is to taste terrible."
– Author Unknown

Back from the funeral, I had more health treatments to undergo. Although I was sad about my granny, I was on a mission. It was time to tackle my parasite issue. In my opinion, everyone has parasites and people with Lyme have MEGA parasites. Just from normal daily living we come into contact with parasites, often unbeknown to us. People who have Lyme disease and other autoimmune diseases have weakened immune systems and have a much harder time thwarting these invaders. The accumulation of parasites often occurs before people even realize it, usually years before an illness prevails.

Bacteria really are parasitic, but knowing that I might also have worms and other types of parasites was enough to make me take the treatment very seriously. I'm sure you can kill worms through conventional medicine. I'm also sure many doctors will tell you it's normal to have them, unless you have overwhelming evidence. Most conventional doctors are not going to look at a dried blood sample or give you a stool test (which only checks for parasites in the gut). Up to this point, I have never had a conventional doctor bring up the parasite issue.

My dried blood analysis (using Darkfield Microscopy) was enough proof for me to do a serious parasite cleanse. Dr. Bob said I had a very bad case and suggested that I use a specific all natural parasite removal kit that kills parasites very effectively (see **Appendix XV** for the kit I take).

The kit takes 30 days to complete. I decided to go full strength (big mistake) and did so for the first two days. Within two days I had Herx reactions on every square inch of my body (red rashes and dots of die-off that burned and were painful to the touch). Some nights, I could barely get into my bed as the pressure of the mattress on my skin caused so much pain. Needless to say, I was so grossed out I could barely speak to anyone or go out in public without covering up. Luckily my face didn't have any Herx rashes (the skin problem started at the neck and went down). I even had to wear flip flops since shoes were too painful to put on.

On the third day the parasite die-off was so intense I had to stop taking the kit for a few days as I was hurting so bad all over and feeling sick. I called Dr. Bob, but since he was having serious ADD problems I could never get him on the phone. The next time I visited, I told him about the ordeal. He said I probably should have taken half strength at first.

I did two kits that year, and I now do a parasite removal once a year (see **Appendix XV**, for more information on parasite cleansing). I've heard of people getting rid of their pets because they fear parasites. I don't think this is necessary. Doing a cleanse once a year takes care of most problems. You can get parasites from your food or eating out. So getting rid of your pet is not going to protect you from parasites. That's a fact. Just make sure your pets get regular de-worming and their medications for fleas and ticks and, obviously, don't kiss your animals on the mouth!

Dr. Bob told me an interesting fact about squirrels, because they don't have parasite problems. They eat the green part of walnuts before they are ripe. The green part kills parasites and I guess instinctively the squirrels know it. Most removal kits that are all natural contain this ingredient (actually called Black Walnut Extract).

By the end of 2007, my parasites were gone. I'd used the energetic medicine (frequency) machines. I'd already made my first trip to the dentist to have the oral pathology cleaned up and I was beginning to feel very well. Toward the end of that year, I started doing some intense physical training again. Even though it was sporadic, it was major progress.

Much of 2007 was spent still working on small, but nevertheless important physical things. I started easy running again. I realized I couldn't just start training "balls to the wall" because I was still in recovery mode. So I started doing more and more physical things and kept seeing Dr. Bob and using the frequency machines. I'd come a long way in a short amount of time, but could tell my body needed to rest. It wasn't that I was still very sick or unhealthy, but the overwhelming need to settle down came over me. I had gotten many of my answers and still felt like there was more to do for some reason. I needed to rest again and regroup my thoughts so I could figure out where I needed to go next.

Chiropractic Care: Finally, Duh!

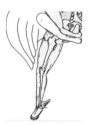

*"It isn't the mountains ahead that wear you out,
it's the grain of sand in your shoe."*
– Author Unknown

After my dental surgery and using Dr. Bob's frequency machines, I realized I was getting closer to getting over Lyme disease with every step because I was always taking steps in the right direction.

Then, in May of 2007, my neck was kind of sore one day while I was driving home from work. I had had a problem with my neck and back ever since my car accident in high school.

I looked again at my thermal image and realized that I had serious inflammation in my back and neck areas. It could be disc-related or it could be simply bacteria-related. Who knew at this point? (Now looking back I believe Lyme travels to areas of the body where it can flourish and this would include areas that are injured or subluxations in the neck or back.)

I decided to get an adjustment. Well, there are good chiropractors and sucky ones, just like in every profession. They all have their own philosophies on how to treat. Fortunately the one I chose made the neck the focus of his practice. He talked me into x-rays, measured my neck from the x-ray and discovered my major structural problem. I had a negative 10 degree curve in my neck. The optimum curve is a 42 degree curve, so I was about 53 degrees off, if you can imagine!

When the neck doesn't curve right, the nerves that run down the spinal column attached to the brain can have a miscommunication when sending messages to the rest of the body because they are not positioned correctly. It made sense. I hadn't had a period since early 2005 when I found out I had Lyme disease. Something was still messed up.

After a week of adjustments, I got my period. After 5 months of neck exercises and getting adjustments, I had a 39 degree curve (not totally perfect but close to it). I had improved 49 degrees in 5 months, and my chiropractor to this day uses my x-rays to show people how amazing progress can be made.

All this time I thought it was Lyme that was keeping me from having my period, but apparently my brain simply wasn't able to communicate with the rest of my body correctly. Our brains are powerful weapons against disease but people don't use it like they should. After making sure the line of communication is clear via the spinal column, using your brain for a specific outcome is incredibly useful. Every time I had treatment like an IV therapy, I would imagine how the solution in the IV was running into my blood, spreading through my body and destroying anything that shouldn't be there. I was imagining the outcome and the usefulness of the treatment.

Athletes do this all the time during competition, and sometimes before a competition they visualize the perfect race or jump or throw or game. They imagine everything in detail from what they sip before they compete, to the sounds they hear while competing. It works. My high school coach always had our team go through a visualizing exercise before a race. I have to give her credit for that one. For a free guided imagery Mp3 on visualizing your recovery and quelling any fears that you may have about your recovery, visit: *www.TheTickSlayer.com/visualize*

Anyone who is ill needs to start visualizing success and what success would be like - down to the things you can physically do and how good you feel doing them. The path from the brain to the spinal column needs to be good (free of subluxations and in alignment) so that the communication is ultra-effective.

Butt Why Not?
Coffee Enemas Anyone?

*"Many great ideas have been lost because the
people who had them could not stand being laughed at."*
– Author Unknown

Recently after reading literature on coffee enemas, I decided to give it a go. Coffee enemas are said to improve the ability of the liver and gallbladder to remove toxins by stimulating the flow of bile and increasing the enzymatic action in the liver to detox.

Although seen as at treatment with no merit, there are plenty of people in the medical world who do believe in their effectiveness. Dr. Nicholas Gonzalez, a controversial figure in the oncology world says, "Coffee enemas help the liver clean out, help eliminate toxic chemicals more efficiently, and make you feel better. Coffee enemas don't destroy bowel function or wipe out your intestinal flora, but what they do is help the liver work better. They are extremely powerful, one of the most powerful detox procedures that we use[1]." Other doctors believe in the effectiveness of coffee enemas, one stating, "They heal the colon, remove many toxins from the liver and colon, often reduce headaches and other body pain, and reduce many symptoms of general toxicity[2]." This common 20th century medical treatment was even added to the Merck Manual, a standard medical reference book from 1899 to 1977.

The coffee enema is, in any case, beneficial just for the ability to increase the glutathione-S-transferases (GST) enzyme. Palmitic acid (a fatty acid) in coffee increases GST, an enzyme involved in detoxification, by 700 times. Coffee also contains theophylline, which increases blood dialysis in the colon by dilating blood vessels.

When mice eat green coffee beans as part of their diet their GST activity increases 600% in the liver and 700% in the small intestine[3]. So why not just drink coffee? Because it's associated with reduced hepatic injury and cirrhosis in humans. Coffee enemas appear to be a more efficient way to get the benefits without getting a caffeine buzz. Most people, even those who tend to get jittery from drinking coffee, report relaxation after a coffee enema[4].

Hopefully the fear of doing an enema the first time, for most people, can be quelled. People who do coffee enemas

1. "Dr. Nicholas Gonzalez On Nutritional Cancer Therapy," The Money Changer, http://the-moneychanger.com/articles_files/health/dr_nicholas_gonzalez.phtml (accessed October 28, 2011).

2. Lawrence Wilson,"Coffee Enemas," http://www.drlwilson.com/Articles/COFFEE%20ENEMA.HTM (accessed September 16, 2011).

3. National Research Council "Diet, Nutrition, and Cancer" National Academy Press; 1982:15-7, 15-8

4. Lawerence, "Coffee Enemas"

usually rave about them. The only precaution I know of is to exercise some restraint when it comes to the number of times you do them each week and to eat something before doing them to avoid hypoglycemic issues. To see the standard procedure on this, please see **Appendix XVI**.

About a year after I tried my first coffee enema I started doing probiotic enemas to keep the integrity of my gut intact by adding in microflora in enormous amounts. I'm convinced that this is the best way to "receive" probiotics and get them to their destination by passing the digestive juices in the stomach. Going the conventional oral route, which is often impaired in people who are ill, only a small percent reaches its intended destination. What I noticed from the probiotic enemas is that I became less sensitive to foods that would sometimes cause digestive issues, my overall health was getting better during this time and I no longer had the dead feeling I used to feel in my solar plexus (which I attribute to my years of eating poorly prior to being diagnosed with gluten-intolerance). The solar plexus sits right above the navel and is a complex network of nerves that intertwines into every organ used for digestion. For more information on these enemas, see **Appendix XVII**.

The Liver Flush

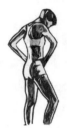

"Symptoms, then, are in reality nothing
but a cry from suffering organs."
– Jean-Martin-Charcot

I knew that my liver had gone through hell up to this point, and I was trying to figure out ways to make it as healthy as possible. For most people who fall ill, a serious focus on liver health is crucial. The QXCI had mentioned that my liver was "overworked and sick," so I kept pressing to find new ways to clean it out and help support it. I was already taking N-acetyl cysteine (NAC for short) and had changed my diet to include more cruciferous vegetables (such as broccoli, cauliflower, brussels sprouts, kale, and cabbage). I had started coffee enemas and had already done an entire colon cleanse. (See **Appendix XVIII** for colon cleansing information.) I was feeling good from all of this, but I had this need to keep going and explore all my options. My mind was certainly open to the wild and whacky as I was having success with my self-treatment and with the suggestions from my encounters with health care professionals and non healthcare professionals alike.

At this time, I was also reading more and more that health is largely dependent on eliminating foreign substances from the body that keep vital organs from performing like they were intended. When I was really ill, I noticed I couldn't sleep through the night without having to pee. It was most annoying (a 26-year-old shouldn't have bladder problems). I felt that perhaps my body was trying hard to get rid of waste and since I had a lot of it, I had to pee every 30-50 minutes when I was really ill (and that meant having to get up constantly at night which made me feel worse because I wasn't getting enough deep sleep to help repair cellular damage). Even people who aren't ill are exposed to a ton of pollutants every day, meaning they too are putting a severe burden on their organs like the liver, colon and kidneys. The coffee enemas were an amazingly cool trick to help the detox process so I thought why not try the liver flush my father had purchased (he got carried away and purchased enough for an entire family to do a flush once a week for an entire year).

There are miles of bile ducts in the liver that can be chock full of cholesterol (which causes cholesterol to rise) and pollutants. The result is what we call a gallstone. When gallstones get too plentiful, the liver makes less bile. It's said that doing a liver flush can help you get rid of these stones, making allergies sometimes disappear and increasing your energy and sense of well-being.

The flush I did consisted of apple juice (organic is best as apples are one of the dirtiest fruits due to pesticides), one cup of olive oil, 1 can of soft drink like ginger ale, juice from a lemon and phosphate drops (see **Appendix XIX** for the type I used). The apple juice and phosphate drops are taken over a few days to saturate the liver. The pectin from the apple and the orthophosphoric acid from the phosphate help soften the stones in the gallbladder and liver. On the last day, you get ready for the flush by mixing the oil, soft drink and the lemon juice and drinking it. The soft drink is optional and is only used so that you don't feel nauseated, but any soda would do. I would prefer a more natural soda that uses organic cane sugar if possible. For days afterwards, if you're like most people, you'll notice green waxy little balls (anywhere from pebble to golf ball size) coming out in your poo. It's a real sight to behold. I had hundreds of these things come out, but I've heard of people who had too many to count.

Because I couldn't hold the oil down, I began vomiting about 1 hr into the "flush" part. I just couldn't handle all of that oil even with the soft drink mixed in. It was dreadful. Now, some people don't get sick from it and it should be noted that many medical professionals think the liver flush is a bunch of phooey, saying that what you're crapping out is actually the oil. I'll let you be the judge of it, but during my recovery my father had an interesting ordeal that could be related to the effectiveness of doing a liver flush.

My father is a real hard ass who eats things he knows he shouldn't and calls me the food Nazi. He suspects he has food allergies (like a self-diagnosed allergy to dairy because of his toilet clinging after eating anything with dairy in it). He also has various medical issues. Yet, he'll go to the doctor and say with a straight face, "I've never felt better. I'm perfectly fine, and I've never been sick in my life." Just a few weeks ago, he was rushed to the ER in an ambulance with a terrible pain in his stomach and gut/liver area. After the routine ER diagnostics, he was discharged and told to see another doctor within a week (which he didn't do). The ER doctors believed he probably had something wrong with his colon or gallbladder, even though they couldn't see anything. (It should be noted that eating the wrong foods alone can give you gallstones.)

My dad had done this liver flush a year earlier but continued with the same "diet."

The next week after his ER trip, my mother made him do another one. This time he pooed out a "stone" the diameter of a 50 cent piece. That could be where the pain was coming from, because if my 173rd Airborne Ranger, Vietnam vet, colonel, attorney dad had to get in an ambulance, you know it had to be AWFUL. He's been okay since but continues to eat whatever and hasn't done the flushes, so I'm sure he'll have some déjà vu in the near future! There are a lot of people out there who swear by the liver flush. I believe the flush is helpful, but shouldn't be done when really ill, as it's tough on the body. Other methods to detox the liver and to support other important organs should be done first.

Some people with Lyme get their gallbladder removed due to this organ becoming severely toxic and dysfunctional. As stated before, I believe the bacteria attacks areas of weakness, so it's important to know that getting your organs healthy (whether it's cleaning them out or taking supplements to support them) is an essential. If the gallbladder ever becomes a problem, ask your healthcare provider to focus on the kidneys and liver, as well as other organs of elimination which directly correlate to the function of the gallbladder.

Back Running Again

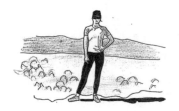

"Do not lose hold of your dreams or aspirations. For if you do,
you may still exist but you have ceased to live."
– Henry David Thoreau

In November of 2007, with the 2008 Olympics on my mind, I felt good enough to start running again. I had been running and doing workouts sporadically for most of 2007, but I knew I couldn't go and really train. In November, the stars must have aligned because I started working out hard and felt really good. I was also confident that I had gotten a lot of my answers and that I was well on my way to completely beating my illness. I didn't know if I was completely healthy or not, but knowing that tests are not that reliable, I skipped them. My symptoms were, I realized, more important than anything. How did I FEEL? The answer was, "pretty good."

It was a far cry from where I was just in the summer of

2005. A year later in the fall of 2006 I was already doing hard runs (but again, it was sporadic). Now it was 2007, and I felt a sense of completion (or close to completion). Since I didn't really know what else I could do at this time and I was feeling good enough to work out hard for a number of days a week, I decided to go back to Florida and give the 2008 Olympics a shot.

I think everyone was a bit surprised at this. Some people had a hard time believing it was the right thing for me to do. Maybe in my mind I always played down the seriousness of the disease. I have never seen myself as a victim, and maybe this was a good thing because I just kept going. You've heard the saying, "love like you've never been hurt before", right? Well, my philosophy is LIVE like you've never been sick before. That doesn't mean going out and ruining your health by partying, staying up late, not listening to your body and constantly putting yourself in stressful situations. It means you have to expect the best, keep going, keep doing the things you love, live your life like you have a second chance.

I packed my things with high hopes, but I decided this time I would do things with far less stress. When I got to Orlando, since this was the first time I had trained in two years, my coach was expecting me to need some serious work. Thankfully, it felt like I never left the sport. Muscle memory is the coolest thing ever. Even though I had lost muscle mass, I was still able to train and run like I had never been sick. About a month into training, however, things stopped going so well.

It wasn't that the Lyme was back. I actually never got a Herx mark again after the end of 2006, no matter what I did to keep trying to kill any Lyme left over in my system. What I didn't realize was that my body needed to recover from the entire ordeal. Even though it had been a long time since I had taken any antibiotics, I was still going through the ramifications! I was only on them for less than 45 days, and that had been 3 years earlier. But I hadn't really given myself a chance to live for a while in sustained good health. My body was in recovery mode, and I was back at it, pushing again. I can say this now, but at the time, I thought maybe I could just take more vitamins and keep going.

I did some looking around and found a doctor in the area and a good chiropractor because my neck was still so sniff that I could barely look over my shoulders when driving while changing lanes. So obviously there were still some things going on.

CRAP!
Integrative Medical Take Two

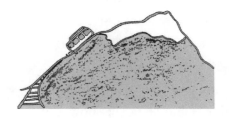

*"It does not matter how slowly you go
so long as you do not stop."*
– Confucius

I did some serious research to find a quality doctor who could get me past the recovery issue. I knew from my experiences exactly what I was looking for. I went to a natural food store and found a free magazine with health info and local services. That was where I found him.

Dr. Kalesh was head of internal medicine at a large hospital in Florida when he became "tired of seeing people die," so he went back to school to get his ND (Naturopathic Doctor) Degree. Dr. Kalesh is also Indian, so he has a good understanding of medicine from other parts of the world (obviously Ayurvedic being one of them, see **Appendix XX** for information on Ayurvedic medicine). This was my kind of guy!

Dr. Kalesh did a consultation with me and had some of his ND interns sit in. After listening to my history, they worked together to create a plan. It was a good plan. The bad news was that it would take about 6 months and I couldn't speed things up. I thought that since it was natural medicine (for the most part), that I could train and it would support me while training But they told me I needed to stop all stressors (including physical stress) to move me in the right direction.

I continued to work out, but my workouts were never done at more than 60% capacity as my coach feared a relapse and knew I was fragile at this point. He must have been terribly impatient with me, but he never showed it.

Dr. Kalesh gave me a video during my first visit with a list of things I needed to start doing. The video was of an Indian man teaching breathing exercises. I learned the exercises and started sun gazing as Dr. Kalesh suggested. Sun gazing is staring directly at the sun with your eyelids closed. The light helps the body heal and stimulates the immune system. There are other gadgets and treatments out there that use the full light spectrum as a way to boost one's immune system.

Dr. Kalesh ordered a bunch of diagnostic tests. He said he suspected that my detox pathways weren't quite functioning optimally. I had told him about the liver detox test done earlier. He wanted me to keep taking N-acetyl cysteine (NAC) to support my own detoxification. I told him I had already put myself on iron, selenium, zinc, D-ribose, essential fatty acids (EFAs) and a whey protein powder (he told me to switch to rice after I told him that it made me feel kind of sick sometimes). Later, I switched to a rice and pea blend (it is a complete protein source without having to take whey). I also started taking Udo's Choice™ for the EFAs, but I found it to be quite nasty. There are other ways to get EFAs, so I eventually had to go to a pill form because just taking a tablespoon of oil was making me queasy. Later, I started taking a tablespoon of extra virgin coconut oil twice a day. It tastes great and has EFAs, in it, something that the QXCI machine at Dr. Bob's was always telling me that I was deficient in. Lastly, he wanted me to take NT Factor, which I had previously been taking.

While waiting for my tests to come back, I started getting a twice-a-week nutritional IV to pump up my suspected depleted levels of multiple nutrients. These multivitamin bags were different from Dr. Rachel's IV vitamin C bags; the formula wasn't just "high" vitamin C. It was now vitamin C; magnesium chloride; potassium chloride; dexpanthenol; cyanocobalamin; B-complex, calcium gluconate; manganese; zinc; chromium; selenium; and folic acid. It worked immediately. I think it was so successful because I hadn't recovered enough and was also trying to get back to my sport. So every time I worked out, I made myself more deficient by using up already low storage levels of necessary nutrients. I just hadn't given myself enough time to recover fully, even though I was well on my way.

Dr. Kalesh has this theory that he calls the web of dysfunction. We all have it. When we get sick, it's because of this web. When you get Lyme disease, your situation is compounded by your prior health problems, no matter how small. So fixing these issues means you can recover; ignoring these issues means you'll stay sick. Here's the breakdown of the web in layman's terms. You have immune system dysfunction (chronic infections, autoimmune diseases and neurological problems). You take antibiotics, steroids or non-steroidal anti-inflammatory drugs (NSAIDS) to try to treat it. You then get candida (a yeast overgrowth that can cause terrible health problems), if you didn't have it before. You also get permeability issues and you might have liver issues now if you didn't already because your liver has been struggling to detox your medications.

This is why people who are sick smell bad. They can't detox and are overloaded with toxins. Leaky gut can add to their food sensitivity issues (one can create the other and both impact each other). Toxins (like heavy metals, pesticides and endotoxins from bacteria die-off) seriously impair your liver and your central nervous system. These neurological effects can create problems with your body making and regulating hormones. So, your adrenals are taxed, your thyroid might not be working right, and your hormones are whacky.

I came to this conclusion before I met Dr. Kalesh, but for the first time I realized someone else got it. During my entire journey he was the most well-versed, all-around doctor I'd seen. I didn't completely know the full ramifications of my situation, but I felt like this was going to be my last stop to a full recovery. I knew these issues had to be addressed. It wasn't Lyme anymore. It was physiological dysfunction from the aftermath. To see explanations of key findings with my standard blood test, see **Appendix IIIb**.

New Therapies

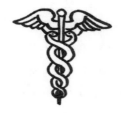

*"Opportunity is missed by most people because it
is dressed in overalls and looks like work."*
– Thomas A. Edison

My micronutrient testing came back showing a deficiency in vitamin D, coenzyme Q-10 and low overall antioxidant function. When fighting an illness like bacteria, it's not uncommon to have low antioxidant levels. My reading was average for the typical person, but I knew I would be at my best as an athlete if I had the desired antioxidant level. I wasn't happy with my results. The test offered repletion suggestions. The multivitamin IV was fantastic, and I also started taking other suggested nutrients, including glutamine (for more information on glutamine, see **Appendix XXII**) because of the suspected damage done to my gut from the antibiotics given by the Lyme specialist, in 2005.

I really have to wonder why infectious disease or Lyme doctors keep putting people on long-term antibiotics. Let's face it; if the tests can be inconclusive and the patient still has symptoms, they could now be sick from processing the die-off of the bacteria and nothing else. The symptoms could also be from the fact that they took a ton of antibiotics, and that people with some type of genetic variance with their liver enzymes might simply be suffering from an overkill of medication and an inability to detox these poisonous substances.

I don't think you can successfully and fully build up someone's immune system if an individual is still taking a pharmaceutical drug, because that means the body is still sick. I keep hearing about Lyme patients who are in their 9th month or 5th year of antibiotics and are still sick, of course they're still sick! *Who wouldn't be?* I'd be half way to hell if I took antibiotics that long (most likely a permanent resident with a parking sticker that lasts for all eternity).

Neurotransmitter Testing

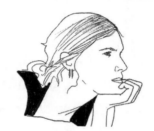

*"Hope is putting faith to work when
doubting would be easier."*
– Author Unknown

D
r. Kalesh also ordered a neurotransmitter test
from NeuroScience, Inc. to test for imbalances
in my nervous system. The test measured urinary
serotonin, dopamine, norepinephrine, epinephrine, GABA,
glutamate, PEA, and histamine. These neurotransmitters
are chemicals that the nervous system uses to send signals
between nerve cells (neurons) as well as to every organ and
tissue in the body to ensure they function properly. They are
directly affected by what we eat, our digestive tract's ability
to break the food down properly and the amount of toxins we
consume as well as their byproducts. Of particular importance
is our liver's ability to carry out its job and filter these toxins.
Approximately 90% of a body's serotonin is made in the
gut and has a strong influence on how the gut breaks down

food[1]. Usually amino acid based supplements are given to correct an individual's nervous system chemistry, but it's important to address nutrition, digestion, and detoxification as well. Laboratory evaluations show that high percentage of the population has some type of neurotransmitter imbalance[2]. Neurotransmitter imbalances can cause depression, fatigue, pain, sleep disorders, irritability, PMS, eating disorders, mood issues, and anxiety[3].

My results indicated that my adrenals were still fatigued and my serotonin was low. I was given two supplements, one that contained 5-HTP which is an amino acid derivative and is used in the synthesis of the neurotransmitters serotonin and melatonin, and one designed to support adrenal function.

It is known that Lyme bacteria can cross the blood-brain barrier. This barrier, part of the circulatory system, is the brain's chemical security system. Neurotransmitters are fat-soluble and do not cross this barrier, but by having the correct load of neurotransmitters, your body can fight the symptoms of this "cross-over of bacteria" because your nervous system is able to send the signals for correction. When people go "nuts" from having Lyme disease, I believe it's partly due to the issues associated with neurotransmitters being unbalanced. Having high levels, for example, causes excessive firing of neurons and disorders like attention deficit disorder (ADD), attention deficit hyperactivity disorder

1. King MW. "Serotonin". The Medical Biochemistry Page. Indiana University School of Medicine. Retrieved 2009-12-01. http://themedicalbiochemistrypage.org/nerves.html#5ht (accessed January 25th, 2012).

2. C Gillberg, "Autistic Children's Hand Preferences: Results From an Epidemiological Study of Infantile Autism," Psychiatry Research (1983) Sept; 10(1):21-30. http://www.ncbi.nlm.nih.gov/pubmed/6580656 (accessed October 21, 2011).

3. King, "Serotonin"

(ADHD), and obsessive compulsive disorder (OCD). Metals, pesticides, some prescription drugs and anti-depressants can cause permanent damage to the nervous system. I believe people on long-term antibiotic "therapy" have a high risk of having permanent damage to their nervous system. Besides these patients constantly have to take new drugs to get at the infection (due to the bacteria becoming resistant), the lasting effects on their nervous system are seen years later. The danger depends on how much is being prescribed, how long someone is on abx (antibiotics) (many medical establishments, including the American Academy of Neurology and the Infectious Disease Society of America, say there is no evidence that taking antibiotics for a prolonged time offers benefit), and of course the type of interaction or the susceptibility to the drug[4]. Most doctors and even Lyme doctors do NOT check a person's liver enzymes to see that person's ability to detox a particular antibiotic. With all the drugs that are being prescribed to people, this is a very bad practice.

Quinolone antibiotics are prescribed in many cases. (Ciprofloxacin is a quinolone that is often prescribed for Lyme disease.) Many people can take a short course of quinolone antibiotics without perceiving any adverse effects. Damage is thought to occur immediately but not enough to create immediate symptoms, because people who are already sedentary can damage joints with repeated short courses and not know it. Later it manifests as osteoarthritis, collagen deterioration, or nervous system failures[5].

4. "New Guideline for Treating Lyme Disease," American Academy of Neurology, news release, May 23, 2007. http://www.aan.com/press/index.cfm?fuseaction=release.view&release=514 (accessed September 16, 2011).

5. T. Boomer, "Quinolone Antiboiotics Toxicity," http://www.antibiotics.org/resources/

There is much debate whether long term antibiotics should or shouldn't be used to treat people with chronic Lyme disease. I have never met a person who had chronic Lyme disease who has said they were completely cured or recovered by taking long term antibiotics and for those people who might think they are cured; I believe that their symptoms will return. With all the toxicity that is involved with taking antibiotics, it just makes sense that over time, lasting effects of the drugs will be seen, if no other major precautions or treatments to diffuse the effects are taken. Unfortunately, because of my journey with this disease, I've met a lot of sick people that I believe are chronically ill due to their prescribed treatment, not the actual disease.

side-effects.pdf (accessed October 2, 2011).

Hormones Evaluated

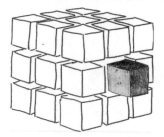

"The part can never be well unless the whole is well."
– Plato

Hormones and neurotransmitters go hand-in-hand (they both affect each other). My hormone panel showed that my cortisol was low and that I had an estrogen dominance (or progesterone deficiency). Taking a natural Progesterone cream was ideal for me. If I wasn't an athlete, I would look into getting Bioidentical Hormone Replacement Therapy; a way of replacing hormones to optimize health. This is a method where hormones are matched to an individual so there is no guessing at what might work. Bioidentical hormones have the same molecular structure as hormones made by our bodies; unlike synthetics which have been made in the laboratory rather than within a biological organism. Bioidentical hormones are thought to metabolized better reducing side effects that can occur with mass produced one-size-fits-all, synthetic hormones, that can produce intolerable side effects. (See **Appendix V** for detailed information on hormone balancing, symptoms associated with an imbalance and why hormones directly affect your health and recovery from illness.)

I had the same test that Dr. Rachel in North Carolina gave me two years prior, to determine my values for TSH, T-4, T3 and cortisol values. All my values had improved and my value for TSH was 2.78, up from 1.76. I wasn't completely fatigued anymore either, but I suspected I still had an underactive thyroid. Although my number was in the normal range, people with hypothyroidism can have normal results and still benefit immensely from getting treated as having an underactive thyroid. See **Appendix IV** for an explanation of hypothyroid conditions and what to get tested.

Getting any thyroid issue resolved will make a lot of people feel better, and anyone who has been sick for a long time will probably have thyroid abnormalities as the body has been in "battle" and the thyroid often becomes a casualty in the war. Thyroid testing should be on every sick person's to do list to help with the fatigue issue that so many people complain about when they are chronically ill.

For my hypothyroid condition, I started taking a drop or two of Lugol's iodine daily as many people with hypothyroid are deficient in iodine. Unfortunately, we just aren't getting the necessary iodine from our foods these days. I also started using mineral salt to cook with that has traces of iodine in it naturally.

Later on I took the same glandular medication that I put my

mother on, one that helps rebuild the thyroid, in addition to a very low level of Armour (a natural from of thyroid hormone from a desiccated thyroid) which I wasn't on for very long, just enough to pump me up while I built up my nutrients to combat the problem naturally. It worked like a charm. Before going on a synthetic, one should always entertain the idea of rebuilding the function of the thyroid through a combination of proper nutrients and a glandular remedy.

Expanded GI Panel

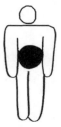

*"From the gut comes the strut, and where
hunger reigns, strength abstains."*
– Francois Rabelais

Because I had told Dr. Kalesh I had a real weakness in my gut at our initial consultation, he was sure I had something wrong with it. He stressed how important the gut's immune system was. I had an expanded GI Panel, so I collected my poo and mailed it in. The test showed I was positive for Cryptosporidium. In immunocompromised individuals that can be severe and even fatal. You can basically get this anywhere; contaminated water is the most common source. The most common immediate symptoms of this are watery diarrhea, stomach pains, cramps and a low fever. However, if left untreated it can cause malabsorption issues, dehydration, leaky gut, ulcers and can even spread beyond the intestines infecting other organs. I also had candida (a very high score). My total SIgA (which is a test to determine the immune strength of my gut) was really low. In fact, this number was 59, and anything below 400 means it's depressed. So my gut was in bad shape. For more information on GI Panels, see **Appendix XXIII**.

I also had a few overgrowths of bacterial pathogens like Streptococcus (I remember this one because the QXCI energy medicine machine months earlier had detected this, but I didn't know what it was at the time) and Corynebacterium (which is RARE, which means I probably got it in Bolivia!). Streptococci bacteria are part of the normal flora in the intestines, but can flourish in people with comprised immune systems. Corynebacterium is a bacteria, commonly found in developing countries, responsible for causing diphtheria (an upper respiratory tract illness), but can also cause extreme infections in the urinary tract. I believe I got this in Bolivia, but because of the language barrier and my incoherent state, I never knew what was given or the diagnosis. After years of living, just about everyone is a walking Petri dish.

Dr. Kalesh gave me a prescription for Alinia™ (Nitazoxanide) to treat the Cryptosporidium because it was potentially deadly. This is why having an ND who is also an MD is very helpful because you get the best of both worlds, someone who believes both in the natural way and in what the Hippocratic Oath really means for doctors (It states: First Do No Harm). Dr. Kalesh whips out the pad when it's the right time to use a prescription, kind of like a last resort for acute deadly infections.

I also started taking a natural candida cleanse three times a day because I still had a major problem with candida yeast that can overgrow due to an imbalance of healthy bacteria in the gut). When the immune system is not working properly healthy gut flora are compromised, usually due to poor diet and use of antibiotics. Candida overgrowth can cause fatigue, anxiety, skin problems, stomach pains, anger outbursts/mood swings, headaches, cravings for sugars, starches and breads, and itchy skin. In really bad cases, candida can also move from the digestive system into the blood stream. (To learn more about candida and how to combat it, see **Appendix XXIV.**)

No wonder I wasn't feeling good. If you feel bad in your gut, it can make you feel bad everywhere!

Bowel Toxemia

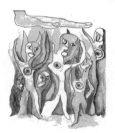

"The body is a community made up of its innumerable cells or inhabitants"
– Thomas A. Edison

When Dr. Kalesh told me how much of our immune system is actually in our gut, I remembered about the QXCI always telling me that I had a "toxic bowel." Sometimes the words on the screen would flash wildly like it was terribly alarmed that I had this. I didn't know at the time exactly how to fix the problem, as this was about 8 months prior to seeing Dr. Kalesh. I did a colon cleanse (with herbs that worked well for me) but if the gut is in really poor shape like mine, much more ammunition is needed. I believe the colon cleanse worked on the physical/mechanical problems, but obviously there were pathogens that still needed to be killed off.

Bowel toxins are the most common toxins in the body.

Starting with the overgrowth of nasty pathogens and partially digested food that sits around and rots (especially animal proteins) accumulating in the gut. These toxins can make people very sick. Obviously, diets high in animal protein and fat and low in complex carbs and fiber contribute to the problem. Bad gut health can lead to what is called bowel toxemia which includes problems like Dysbiosis (a fancy name describing when the pathogens are too numerous in the gut, causing chronic indigestion). Some common symptoms of this imbalance are poor digestion, rheumatoid arthritis, spastic colon, itchy anus, hypoglycemia, body odor, bad breath, flatulence, bloating, colon cancer, constipation or diarrhea, and abdominal pains.

Our neurotransmitters are directly affected by our digestion and our liver's ability to detox. Some of the physical symptoms include: headaches, sciatica, fatigue, nervousness, impaired nutrition, skin problems, hormone problems, low back pain, allergies and eye, ear, nose and throat problems. It doesn't mean that all of the problems come directly from the bowels, but bowel toxemia is almost always overlooked as a big contributing factor. People who go to a chiropractor without any relief from their low back pain or thoracic subluxations should probably get their gut checked.

It's easy for pathogens to take over when the gut is so unhealthy (and Lyme is a pathogen). Since around 75% of our body's total immune system is in the gut, we can boost our immunity by improving our gut health.

Some ways to treat bowel toxemia are extended juice fasts (which provide rest to the overworked bowels, allowing inflammation to subside, but should not be done by those who are weak and already depleted), changes in diet (less animal protein, fat and refined food and more complex carbs, fruits and vegetables), avoiding overeating, taking care to consume the largest meal in the afternoon, not at night when digestive energy is low, exercise and re-colonizing the intestines with a probiotic supplement.

Obviously for me to get my gut health back, I had to go a step further because I had to repair my gut from antibiotic damage as well as lingering pathogens. I started by taking glutamine, massive probiotics (in the billions with many different quality strains) and a product containing gamma-linolenic Acid (borage seed oil), gamma-oryzanol and phosphatidylcholine. (see **Appendix XXV** for more information.)

Working on my gut health has made a remarkable difference in the fatigue that I've had for years while running and racing. I never thought I had a problem because I was hardly ever constipated. That's the one symptom that lets someone know the gig is up! Runners actually tend to have diarrhea (especially before races) from nerves, but I'm guessing others have ticking time bombs in their guts. Visiting a port-a-potty before a road race should be avoided at all costs!

I also started drinking ozonated water and using it for enemas. (Ozonated water contains 03, which is a more volatile molecule of oxygen.) Ozone has many applications for its cleaning ability. Ozone is produced naturally in the body by white blood cells as a way of killing pathogens in the blood and has been used as a treatment for various ailments. The danger with ozone comes from the fact that when taken internally, either through inhalation or IV, it can create free radicals. On the flipside, it is being used medicinally in countries that are progressive in treating disease. Cancer cells, for example, die when exposed to oxygen and many healthcare professionals believe that all disease comes from oxygen deficiency. Therefore, increasing oxygen in one's system can be health promoting.

I've never, to this day, had complications from using ozone, nor have I heard of anyone getting sick from ozone use. The enemas are no more uncomfortable than using plain water and when drinking ozonated water there is no detectable difference from drinking plain water. I believe that just the use of ozone in my daily life has kept my susceptibility to various infections (including respiratory) and intestinal parasites very low.

Ozone machines are used as air purifiers, as a means to remove pesticides from foods, as a way to launder clothes, or to kill bacteria in hot tubs or pools, just to name a few well known applications. (To find out more about ozone therapy and machines for home use See **Appendix XXVI**)

Parasites, worms, fungus, mold, yeast and bacteria cannot live in an oxygen-enriched environment. After doing this quick enema, I noticed some very unsightly spaghetti-type, blobs of worms coming out. I had been feeling fatigue in my lower legs for the entire week, and the day after this enema, my leg power was back. So instead of going "that's gross," you should probably turn your attention to your unwanted visitors. Everyone has worms!

In the USA, one-third of about 6,000 fecal specimens tested at PCI were positive for 19 species of intestinal parasites[1]. According to the Center for Disease Control, an

---

1. Omar M Amin, "Seasonal Prevalence of Intestinal Parasites in the United States during 2000," American Journal of Tropical Medicine and Hygiene, 66(6):799-803).

estimated one-third of the entire world's population has an intestinal parasite, and it's well known that the CDC reporting is always on the low end[2]. Many parasites are so well adapted the host can be entirely asymptomatic. The reason for the large number of infected people could be because of increased travel, increased contamination of the water and food supply and the overuse of chemicals, mercury and prescription antibiotics. Parasites are found in the highest concentration in commercial pork products (bacon, ham, hot dogs, cold cuts, pork chops, etc.).

2. CDC, "Domestic Intestinal Parasite Guidelines", http://www.cdc.gov/immigrantrefu-geehealth/guidelines/domestic/intestinal-parasites-domestic.html (accessed September 14, 2011).

Urine Toxic Metals Test

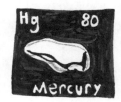

"The only thing wrong with doing nothing is that you never know when you're finished."
– Author Unknown

M etals are in everyone, but high levels can lead to impairment of your body's natural mechanisms. I had a urine loading test done to determine my levels. The way this test works is that you get an IV containing a solution that binds with the metals. Then you do a urine loading sample where you collect your urine for a number of hours to get an average. This sample then goes to the lab. You can also get a hair analysis done to see how high your metals are. See **Appendix XXVII** for more information on testing.

I had no metals from dentistry so that was one plus on my side. But still, I had elevated levels of mercury, as well as lead and aluminum. I was also slightly elevated for nickel.

Since the solution that adheres to the metals made me feel

like crap, I didn't chelate the metals until months later as Dr. Kalesh didn't think it was the main issue. Plus, the bound metals going through my gut to be defecated and urinated out was stirring up the pathogens. So it was better to treat the gut first. These agents that are used to chelate metals (see **Appendix XXVII** for more information) also remove nutrients like essential minerals, so having your levels of nutrients balanced before and during the chelating process is vital.

Mercury detoxification (as well as detoxifying from other metals) is thought to be a very good treatment against Lyme disease or any autoimmune disease simply because mercury toxicity often accompanies these diseases. The two illnesses certainly impact each other. Mercury weakens the immune system and perhaps by doing so, makes people more susceptible to illness (like Lyme disease). Lyme disease, on the other hand, weakens the body's ability to detox various substances, making a person more susceptible to accumulating a poison like mercury.

Driving On

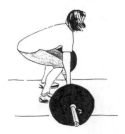

*"Before a diamond shows its brilliancy and
prismatic colors it has to stand a good deal
of cutting and smoothing."*
– Author Unknown

Now all this testing and treatment took some time, about 5 months. The first plan included the nutritional IVs (which included the B12 and folic acid because my blood test indicated the deficiency), the attack on the yeast in my gut, Co-Q10 to pump up my cellular energy, vitamin D to cover that deficiency, a strong probiotic, two supplements for my neurotransmitters and exhausted adrenal glands, an Alinia prescription for the Cryptosporidium in my gut, and the glutathione push to pump up this important free-radical scavenger that I was terribly deficient in. I also stayed away from soy and gluten since I knew for sure those were two foods my body could not tolerate.

The second plan of attack included D-ribose and NT

Factor again to pump up my cellular energy. At this time my only real complaint was my energy and a stiff neck, which I would later attribute to the infection in my mouth that was still draining. (I had yet to realize that the surgery I had done in Tennessee did not get all of the infection out, so it became re-infected and was keeping me ill.)

Dr. Kalesh, unaware of the dental connection, focused on treating other metabolic issues, and suggested milk thistle and castor oil presses to help me detox my liver. Castor oil presses involve rubbing castor oil over your liver area, putting piece of clean cloth like a towel on top of the oil and then using heating pad to warm the area.

I think the milk thistle was more beneficial. The thistle is not only useful it's actually a very well known Scottish emblem. The thistle plant thrives in harsh conditions, suggesting endurance and fortitude (you could say it's a real bastard of a plant).

The use of this herb helps protect the liver against toxicity and helps regenerate the liver by stimulating the growth of liver cells. Milk thistle is very well researched herb and is best noted for its use to improve liver function against liver cirrhosis and other serious liver diseases like Hepatitis. With all the drinking Scots and Irish do, they should not only wear it, but also take it. Dr. Kalesh wanted me to do both treatments as he suspected from the blood test results that my liver was in really bad shape, so I was attacking the problem with multiple strategies.

Russian Doctor and Aerophytotherapy

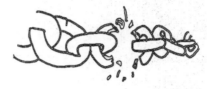

*"If the truth be known, most successes are built
on a multitude of failures."*
– Author Unknown

D r. Kalesh suggested I work with one of his colleagues who had been studying Lyme disease and treating people with aerophytotherapy, a treatment using high quality essential oils to kill Lyme by inhalation. Little did I know that years earlier, I had read research that she had conducted.

After giving her my history, Dr. Valora asked me about where I grew up. I told her about living in the country and running around playing in the woods half-naked all day. She was the first doctor to tell me that having the Lyme disease hallmark, bull's-eye rash, was a sign that I had already contracted the disease before I was bitten in 2003. She said that I more than likely got it as a child. It was activated from my car accident with the bus my last year in high school, making me suffer in college with fatigue and be more susceptible to other viruses like Epstein-Barr virus. It all made sense. I was kind of relieved someone helped me put it together, even though it didn't mean that I would treat anything differently, but it gave me answers that I wanted and needed.

Dr. Valora's therapy using essential oils was interesting. I sat in a sealed room infused with an essential oil blend. Sometimes, while breathing in the oils, I would get numb in my face and gut, but most noticeably in my gut area. Dr. Valora had done the research and concluded that you can kill Lyme and strengthen the immune system through this therapy. I had about 8 sessions, but because I felt like I was still putting a band aid on a gaping wound, I stopped and kept looking for that BIG answer. I knew in my heart something was not right and was keeping the therapy from working better.

Answers from Strange Places

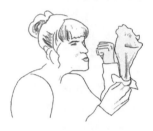

*"Successful men follow the same advice
they prescribe for others."*
– Author Unknown

People who are totally "nuts" in one way or another can be extremely beneficial (some would say dangerous), especially when they are in the health arena. I had the fortune of meeting lots of them during my journey and am grateful for every encounter. I found that most were self-educated, some had their PhDs, some were chemists and some were researchers. While under the care of Dr. Kalesh, I had a phone conversation with a good friend of mine whom I had met earlier through Dr. Bob. She told me that I should go see a guy in Virginia who was really far out there, trying to do new things with healthcare. She suggested him because I was a little down about taking all these medicines and treatments and having months of recovery still ahead of me. I was lying to myself at this time, thinking I could hurry it up and keep training. I was still wondering why my energy was so poor and my neck was so stiff (even though I was getting regular chiropractic care in Orlando for maintenance).

I called this man whom I'd never met and explained the situation he told me to pack my bags and get up to see him quickly. He had many gadgets for me to play with and during February in snow-covered central Virginia, I unlocked my last medical mystery.

Joe was a massage therapist by profession but he was also a self- made millionaire as he dabbled in all kinds of businesses. His house contained piles of every health gadget known to man. You could say he was a health enthusiast, but the extent of his formal training was massage school.

Joe liked to use his hands as, "instruments of God" to heal people. He once told me about this woman who was very sick, and while he was working on her one day, he asked God to help him heal her. He said his hands got red, and the woman was healed in an instant. Okay, so I have a very hard time believing that, but these days I can't not believe something just because I didn't see it. So I remain neutral on the subject.

Joe's Gadgets

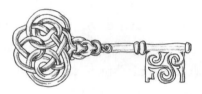

"Don't be discouraged. It's often the last key in
the bunch that opens the lock."
– Author Unknown

Sweat contains more toxins than urine. Sweating is a powerful healing tool, as the skin is an organ that removes waste (sometimes called the 3rd kidney). Ever wonder why Native Americans have their sweat lodges and often use them to heal themselves of strange illnesses? Sweating enough can actually help you remove heavy metals! Some other health benefits of sweat therapy are: increased blood circulation, prevention of colds, skin rejuvenation, pain reduction for arthritis, increased energy, body detoxification, healing of sore muscles, stress relief, weight loss, and a stronger immune system.

Joe introduced me to his first gadget, the Infrared Sauna (a sauna that uses infrared heat (dry heat) to bake you).

I bumped up the heat to 126 degrees and gave it a go for an hour. I still wasn't having any Herx symptoms so while this helped me detox, I got confirmation again that the Lyme wasn't the real issue anymore. I had two sessions in his sauna, but to be honest, my hot car sauna worked just as well in the summertime (due to the intense heat in the Carolinas).

I called the next gadget I used, "The Pod" because it's a large plastic capsule that only your head sticks out of as you sit inside on a towel. Your body gets steam-blasted with ozone. If you have metals, they can often come out in your sweat, most visible as tiny black sand-like granules if you sit on a white towel during a session. The Pod is torture. It made my body so hot that I was sweating buckets and was thankful my face was not inside the capsule; however, I can see the benefit in it. After all, you pee it out, poop it out, breathe it out or sweat it out. I give it an A+ for detoxing and getting the waste out of my lymph nodes. (For information on the sauna pod and how these gadgets work, see **Appendix XXVIII**.)

Yet another one of Joe's gadgets wasn't fancy at all, it was a mini trampoline. Joe was telling me about using it as a way to strengthen my lymphatic system. Often called "rebounding," this is an exercise that gets the valves in the lymphatic system to open and close simultaneously, increasing the flow of lymph fluid (which flows in the direction opposite to gravity). People with chronic disease have stagnant lymph fluid which becomes a haven for viruses, bacteria and other pathogens. Our lymph system runs through our entire body and contains fluid that sends nutrients to cells and carries the waste products away. The lymphatic system is totally dependent on physical exercise; therefore it's a must that one keeps moving to stay healthy.

The best part about rebounding is that it's easy and you don't even have to jump, you just bob up and down. I started doing it 15-20 minutes each day, and still use it as a way to stay healthy. For more information on rebounders, visit: *www.TheTickSlayer.com/rebound*

Other ways to improve lymphatic congestion include consuming enough water on a daily basis along with a teaspoon of Himalayan salt and getting lymphatic massage done. There is also a device called a LBG and/or ST-8 that can penetrate deeper than massage to restore lymphatic movement. This cutting edge technology "do-no-harm" modality helps with revitalization and detoxification. To see how the LBG works in detail, visit: *www.TheTickSlyaer.com/LBG*

Lastly, Joe wanted to show me his ozone gadget called he created. The lymph nodes around my neck were swollen and my neck hurt. Joe made this gadget that looked like a wand that dispensed ozone (O3) onto my skin where it was absorbed. Joe worked on me for about 30 minutes with the wand and then said "I'm not going to tell you how I do this, but I have O15. It's super potent oxygen, and I call it the Breath of God." He told me to take a swig of it after he pulled a container of it out of his refrigerator. I took a swig and used it like mouthwash.

A few seconds later, I had blood coming out my nose but it was not bright red blood like a nose bleed, instead it had the look of infection. I had never had a sinus infection so I was worried. But I realized that when anything unwanted, like bacteria or infection, comes into contact with something like O15 or even O3, it causes a reaction. O3 and higher forms of unstable oxygen can neutralize harmful organic material such as viruses, bacteria and other pathogens. It acts as a cleaning agent, but can cause a surge of free radicals depending on how much harmful material there really is. I knew the strange material coming out of my nose was more than likely my body trying to shed itself of infection still left in my jaw.

I had a hunch that these sites were not completely cleared out, but this sealed the deal in my mind. I knew that the tissue surrounding my jaw and cartilage in my face is all connected, the infection was still there and that was why the blood was coming out of my nose.

Joe finished up by trying to do some healing on me, but I got no miracles. So I thanked him profusely for opening his home to me and sharing his equipment and went back to Orlando to make some calls and find another dentist! I knew what I had to do, but I was so upset on the flight back. I felt that I was so close but here was something else again--and the worst part was that I thought I had already jumped over this hurdle. I had to have surgery AGAIN.

The Final Push

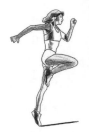

"I will neither yield to the song of siren nor the voice of the hyena, the tears of the crocodile nor the howling wolf."
– George Chapman

My coach told me I had 15 weeks before the Olympic Trials. Coach knew that my success was largely dependent on my health. He knew that I could do everything I wanted to athletically if I was healthy, so he pretty much stayed out of my way while I was taking care of things. When I told him I had to have surgery again he was, for the first time, visibly upset. He knew at that moment I wouldn't be going to the trials. I was still hoping for the best, thinking that I could get it taken care of ASAP and keep going. After all, I felt good after the first surgery (I drove three and a half hours to get back home because I felt so great). I had high hopes, but I should have taken my cue from Coach. Sometimes when you're so mentally invested in something it's hard to let go. During this journey back to health, I got really good at letting go of everything.

Back in Orlando from my revealing visit to Virginia, I called my friend again. She was from California and was very knowledgeable about oral pathology. Years earlier her regular dentist left an impacted tooth in her mouth that later became infected. Her face was swollen from the infection which became life threatening. The problem for her was that no one knew how to treat it since the infection was basically in the entire left side of her face. Once a tooth is infected or a cavitation is infected, it's just a matter of time before the jaw and all of the connective tissue in the face rots and/or leaks toxic infection that travels to other areas of the body causing disease.

She told me that she had gone on the same journey as I had, except hers was solely because of her dental problem. She told me about all her "adventures", stupid doctors and, of course, the doctors who became her saviors. These saviors for her were actually dentists, biological dentists.

I told her that I had to know who the best biological dentist was, explaining how upset I was about the infection still being there. She told me a little bit about how the same situation played over and over for her as well. Her case, however, was much worse than mine. Yes, I had Lyme disease on top of it, but her pathology was bringing her to her knees, all because of one incompetent dentist.

She told me to go to Houston, Texas, to see Dr. Glaros for these matters. I was on the plane the next day. I thought if I could get it done, I would still have time to get ready for the 2008 Olympic Trials. But the weeks were counting down, and I didn't have a moment to spare.

The Beginning of the Very End

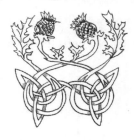

May God give you...
For every storm, a rainbow,
For every tear, a smile,
For every care, a promise,
And a blessing in each trial.
For every problem life sends,
A faithful friend to share,
For every sigh, a sweet song,
And an answer for each prayer.
– Irish Prayer

I had done a pretty fantastic job attacking Lyme disease and getting most of my health back. I could certainly function as a normal person, but I knew to be an athlete, I had to be 100%, and I wasn't going to settle for anything less. I wanted this infection out of my mouth! I flew into Houston, rented a car, drove a few miles and went straight to my appointment (it was a whirlwind trip). I was excited and ready to move on!

I first met with a Naturopathic Doctor who worked with Dr. Glaros, the dentist. I couldn't believe he worked with a naturopath (this is rare), and I felt relieved because I knew he checked his ego at the door so I was already liking this guy. The naturopath took some MSA/EAV (Meridian Stress

Assessment and Electro Acupuncture) readings of each tooth in my mouth with a type of ElectroDermal Screening (EDS) device. (ElectroDermal Screening devices are the invention of Dr. Reinhardt Voll[1].) Most people don't realize that each tooth has a meridian that specific organs are associated with. If a certain tooth is decayed, the coordinating organs can be affected negatively. In addition to each tooth being tested, certain acupuncture points on my hand were also tested.

From this machine, in conjunction with a Cavitat, dental x-rays, a panoramic x-ray, this dentist knew where I still had infection with less guessing and more precision.

The dentist in Tennessee had successfully cleaned one cavitation, out of four that were in question, without re-infection occurring. So I had two places where surgery had to be performed again, and one place that was never operated on in the first place and should have been! All four wisdom tooth extractions left infected cavitations and had to be cleaned. This type of incident is exactly why healthcare professionals should incorporate all technology and sciences when trying to heal people. Had the surgery been done right the first time around, I would have been in Beijing in 2008 eating with chopsticks.

I knew I was in good hands with these people in Texas and was relieved to be there. I can't explain my joy, even though I knew I was going to be in serious pain later, I didn't care.

Dr. Glaros, the dentist, came in and spoke to me while his assistant was prepping me for surgery. We both had Nikes on; I felt like this was a good sign. Probably even a better sign was that this guy valued my opinion. He asked me questions,

1. Voll R., "New Electroacupuncture (EAV) measurement points for various eye structures." Amer. Journal of Acupuncture. March 1979

and really listened to my answers. We spoke about the disease situation and about other people who had the same thing going on.

Cavitation cleanup is an outpatient surgery done while the patient is awake. Local anesthesia is used to numb specific areas. Unfortunately I had the same problem with the Xylocaine® as I did in Tennessee with the Novocain, I was so busy fighting Lyme and taking high doses of vitamin C that it was making me detox the Novocain too quickly! I had stopped taking vitamin C a week before the surgery, but apparently it wasn't enough time for my body to completely flush the excess C. I was at my legal limit for Xylocaine for my body weight and it was time to do the Epinephrine. The limits of safe administration levels of anesthesia are related to the anesthetic itself and not the level of vasoconstrictor.

A homeopathic remedy of the local anesthetic was created by putting a drop of each kind of anesthetic in four ounces of bottled water. The solution was then put in my mouth and amazingly, I had no problems with the Epinephrine this time!

Dr. Glaros spent all afternoon with me. He lightly drilled a hole to tap into my cavitation pockets and then scraped the diseased bone out. I had the "black oil" come out again. The scraping was so aggressive that the assistant had to hold my head steady. I was kind of freaking out, so I just looked at the poster of a pretty forest hanging on the ceiling and hummed show tunes (which Dr. Glaros tried to guess as he was working). We played this game for hours, during the parts of the surgery that weren't so intense. If he was totally annoyed by it, he sure didn't show it.

I felt like I could go for a run during the surgery, probably because the infection was being removed. I started humming the theme song from *Rocky* and telling his naturopath to "get all of that crap out," which I'm not sure she understood with all of the dental tools in my mouth. While my sites were still open, Dr. Glaros called in his naturopath and she used the EDS device to probe the cavitations to see if Dr. Glaros had gotten everything. They checked 5-8 times, until they got the same clean reading from slightly different points. Then they knew that it was time to close up.

Dr. Glaros closed the sites, compressing the tissue over the site covering it so that the gum tissue could be in intimate contact with the bone, bubble-less and ready to heal. Keeping the soft tissue out of the bone socket allows the boney material to grow back to replace the diseased bone of a cavitation site. When Dr. Glaros was finished, the ND took part of the removed infection out and created a homeopathic solution that I was to take under my tongue every fifteen minutes. The post surgical drops (a homeopathic nosode that contained part of the diseased material.) were made specifically for me and were to accelerate my post-surgical recovery. I was also given a piece of Silverlon® cloth, a fabric with sliver thread woven into it, to be placed near the surgery site to help reduce swelling and pain and to keep bacteria away. A predigested protein supplement containing amino acids, minerals and omega 3 fatty acids from white fish, was to be taken daily. It provided protein that required no digestion, and since I wasn't going to be able to eat for a while, it was a great nutrient to take. Amino acids help build healthy tissue and assist in the recovery of surgery sites. Lastly, Nattokinase (also called Natto, see **Appendix XXIX** about the importance of Natto, how it was developed and the common uses for it.) was given to help improve the blood flow to the surgery site.

Dr. Glaros and I had a little chat at the end, and he said it would take 6 months to a year for those cavitations to heal completely. It didn't mean I would be sick for months afterwards. It just meant that since the heart of the infection was removed, the other connective tissue, bone, etc. would finally heal overtime. Part of why I felt a little icky when working out hard and why my neck was still so stiff was simply because this infection was still "dripping" into my immune system, keeping my body in a constant state of high alert. The lymph nodes in my head and neck were taking the brunt of the "leaking" infection. After the surgery I had to ask his dental assistant how bad it was. She said one cavitation was about an 8 out of 10.

The lady at the front desk asked if I wanted a few pain killers before I left. Since I had a prescription I would have to get filled, I said no because I felt fine. I hopped into my rental car, and as I was driving to my hotel a few miles away, the anesthesia wore off in a flash! I wasn't familiar with the area and partly because I was drugged I couldn't figure out how to get back to the dentist's office. To make things worse, the pain was intensifying rapidly and dramatically. Dr. Glaros had scraped around root nerves, and I was getting ready to experience the worst pain I had ever felt in my life.

I drove to find a place to fill my prescription ASAP because I was wigging out and crying from the searing pain. I knew if I didn't get help soon, I would pass out. I was on the interstate in rush hour traffic in Houston looking desperately for a pharmacy, barely able to drive. (Warning: Don't do what

I did. First, have someone go with you to the surgery to drive you. Second, take pain killers BEFORE you leave the office.) Finally, I spotted a Walmart and ran in, saying "Please help, I have to have my prescription." I must have looked like an addict; because that's the look the lady behind the counter gave me.

I explained quickly that I had just had dental work done (my face was "only" half swollen on both sides) and that I was in enough pain to pass out on the floor. I was shaking and almost crying. The lady told me that I had to wait in line because, I guess, Grandma who was there before me needed her glaucoma prescription first. I had to take a number. After 15 minutes and more violent shaking, I asked how much longer, and she said she didn't know. I was dangerously close to passing out or fighting the pharmacist like a wild, caged animal. Anything could have happened at that moment.

I turned around and ran out the door, got into my car and floored it out of the parking lot like a maniac! I soon found a drug store and ran in. There were a few people waiting, but the girl at the counter was sympathetic, as her mom had dental work a few days earlier. She had the prescription filled in less than 2 minutes. I thanked her graciously, ripped it open and took one right away. I walked around in the store, drying my tears before I felt it was safe to get in my car again to go find a hotel.

The hotel closest to the dentist's office was booked, but honestly at this point I probably wouldn't have been able to find it even if I had reservations. So I ended up at the first motel I found. It was the type of motel where the rooms open up from the outside, and as I drove in, I was totally unaware what a crap hole it really was. I got the key-card to my room and drove around back to my room, passing truckers hanging out in their doorways. They were looking like a bunch of 10 cent hookers (actually it probably would have been free) and being partially drugged was making me even more uncomfortable. I hoped that they were a bunch of gay truckers. A few men were standing in their doorways, shirtless; rubbing their bellies and when they went into their rooms, I got out of my car and ran into my room. I didn't leave my room again that night.

The medication was just enough to take the edge off, but I felt terrible pain everywhere. I was detoxing hard and even though the heart of the infection was out, some of it had been released freely into my immune system during the surgery. I ran to the bathroom but didn't want to throw up because I didn't want to get vomit into my surgery sites. I couldn't contain it though. When the yellow bile substance was vomited out it was mixed with part of that "black oil" that drained out of my cavitations during surgery. I ran a hot bath to try to take the pain away and get my body temperature up. I couldn't control it and began to shake all over and my lips started to turn purple. Anyone who saw me that evening probably thought I was a heroin addict who couldn't get a fix! I looked terrible, and struggled to take care of myself the best way I could. I was prepared with juices, teas, soups I could make by heating (my own clean) water in the coffee pot. I also brought various supplements, because I had had an idea of what was in store for me with this surgery.

The next day I felt like I had been hit by a bus and the pain in my mouth had only subsided by about 20%. Not enough for me to get home comfortably, but my flight was leaving and I didn't want to stay another night in that hotel. I would never attempt to do something like this by myself again, but I had no idea the surgery would be so aggressive. The prior surgery basically drained the infection, and I never suffered from the removal of the actual decayed bone matter. To get more information about this process, see **Appendix 2-I**, for details from Dr. Glaros.

Flying back home was interesting. Never have I had so many strangers pity me. I never had to say a word. I guess I looked bad enough. My hair was a mess, but I didn't realize how swollen my face was until I used the bathroom at the airport. The good news is that my stewardess was super attentive, and I appreciated it. When I got back to Orlando, it looked like I had eaten two tennis balls and the lymph nodes around my neck looked like golf balls. I was still in severe pain, but part of me was relieved to finally have this lingering issue resolved. I could finally move on to a full recovery and go back to track, even if it wasn't meant to be that year.

The Final Recovery

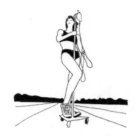

*"If people knew how hard I work to get my mastery,
it wouldn't seem so wonderful at all."*
– Michelangelo

B ack in Orlando, I could barely take care of myself.
I finally had to give in and ask my mother to come
out and help me.

I was yacking every 30 minutes for 2 days straight.
Infection after infection after infection just came pouring out
of my mouth. It was a puke fest that would put any bulimic
pizza party to shame. I felt so bad just sitting around, so I
started to skin brush (taking a brush specifically made to brush
the skin in order to release toxins trapped by your skin) and
rebound to get my lymph nodes to remove the waste quicker.
I felt so toxic I wanted to die, so I brushed and jumped, and
every time I did, I had to run quickly to the bathroom and
puke more infection out!

In order for bacteria like Lyme to survive treatment it can hide in the lymphatic system, clogging it. Lyme is a systemic infection, so it travels everywhere (including into cavitations in the mouth). The enormous swelling of my lymphatic system and my severe pain was, I believe, my Lyme's last hoorah. It was hanging on for dear life, and I wasn't letting up on my side either.

I couldn't sleep lying down because the lymph nodes in the back of my head were so swollen. I started sleeping sitting up in bed to help move the waste out of my head area (I was also having vertigo/pressure issues).

Finally 72 hours passed and the weekend was over. On Monday I called Dr. Glaros. I have never called a doctor for an emergency, but in this case I was wondering if my ordeal was normal. He said it was for some people, depending on the severity of the infection in the mouth (damn, mine must have been really bad). I felt too weak to go see Dr. Kalesh and get the nutritional IV, which I knew would help me flush this out. On Tuesday I rallied and spoke to Dr. Kalesh. He said I could take Welchol® (if I wanted). Welchol (colesevelam hydrochloride) binds to infection and pulls it out, but it's mainly a drug for people with high cholesterol. I thought about it, but the nutritional IV was doing a pretty bang up job pumping me back up. I never took the Welchol, but I probably should have as I could have used another method to absorb all the toxicity I was overloaded with. There are probably numerous factors to why the aftermath of my surgery was so horrendous and this does not illustrate a typical procedure. I just had a seriously infected jaw, filled with a lot of nasty things (insert frowny face).

What was really comical is that 4 days after I returned from my surgery, I decided to go to practice because time was ticking. Our strength trainer asked me if I had lost some weight (which was a nice way of saying, "you look like shit"). I said "of course, I can't eat!" saying this with my mouth slightly closed due to the stitches. I felt like crap and had to stop running. It wasn't going to work. The initial hell week of recovery had severely depleted me. A few weeks later, I was done throwing up…finally! I started to try some new immune system treatments because I felt like it was needed.

Free Radical Overload

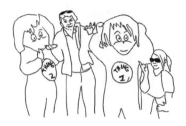

*"If there are obstacles, the shortest line between
two points may be a crooked line."*
– Bertolt Brecht

I knew from my blood test that my antioxidant level was pretty average, but not good enough to combat the stress my body was going through. I knew I was suffering from free radical overload (free radicals are atoms with unpaired electrons and can be formed when oxygen interacts with certain molecules). The surgery had left my immune system fighting off any last pathogens (including Lyme bacteria and co-infections) left in my jaw bone. So neurotoxins were coming into play once again.

Neurotoxins create free radicals and lead to oxidative stress, causing all kinds of health damage. There are two ways to combat this; one, getting more antioxidants, which I was doing through the multivitamin IVs and the glutathione injections (major protective antioxidant). The other is by increasing the oxygen in the body. Increased oxygen enables mitochondria (cells that create energy) to energize neurons.

I think free radical overload is probably quite common even if someone is seemingly healthy. We live in times when pollution is so common and many of us are oblivious to the dangers. We use products full of chemicals, our food is contaminated with pesticides and herbicides, and our tap water is chlorinated and never as pure as it should be. Because of these issues, my liver still needed TLC (Tender Love and Care) and so did my gut. I had to restore my health via these two major organs, while boosting oxygen to these tissues and getting enough antioxidants to combat the free radicals.

The most prominent neurotoxin associated with Lyme disease is ammonia. Because a sick or overloaded liver cannot convert it, ammonia can build up and pass through the blood-brain barrier. I remember Dr. Bob in North Carolina telling me about a man sick with cancer who stunk of ammonia and was on the verge of dying. He told me that he was able to detox the man of the ammonia/aldehyde, prolonging his life for several more years. Apparently, neurotoxins (which are nerve poisons) are understood to be the number one cause of symptoms experienced by people suffering from Lyme disease, degenerative disease and cancer!

Molybdenum is a trace mineral that can be helpful with detoxing neurotoxins, and even yeast (candida) die-off. Beta-Sitosterol is also helpful and is a phytosterol with a chemical structure similar to cholesterol that comes from a plant-based phytochemical. If I could go back, I would have taken these supplements throughout my ordeal.

In addition to the nutritional IVs and glutathione pushes, I started eating wheat grass, barley grass and alfalfa sprouts. These foods are loaded with essential vitamins, minerals and amino acids. I also craved foods rich in antioxidants like berries, nuts, beans, leafy green vegetables, and teas. I became a total fiend for yerba mate (a South American root with a very high ORAC value that is made into a tea). You might see the letters ORAC on food packages. It stands for Oxygen Radical Absorbance Capacity. It's the ability of that food to scavenge free radicals, so the higher number the better!

Inflammation Damage Control

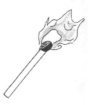

"The biggest bonfire starts from the smallest spark."
– Richard Saunders

I often hear people complain about inflammation in the joints, including most people with Lyme disease. Many have Rheumatoid Arthritis, or it is in the making. Rheumatoid Arthritis is just inflammation, and obviously inflammation in the joints is as damaging as it is in the gut. I had tell-tale signs of inflammation everywhere in my body. The pain in my gut and other areas may have been so severe that I overlooked everything else. My stiff neck that could not be cured by chiropractic care went away after I had my visit to the biological dentist in Texas. I believe that reducing the waste products in the body by detoxing, quenching the inflammation, and strengthening and oxygenating the tissues in the joints is a pretty fail-proof plan.

A friend of mine, years prior, told me about an aloe that was specially processed so that it was enzyme-enriched and so concentrated that a tablespoon had more power than an entire bottle of the aloe juice sitting on the shelves at super markets. I started taking the concentrate because I craved it. Aloe has been known to heal just about every kind of condition known to man. In Egypt it was a prized plant and used for a wide range of ailments. I was using it for its antioxidant properties and polysaccharides that could help heal damaged tissue. Strong doses of aloe have also have been purported to cure gut problems, because of its ability to quench inflammation and to repair damage on a cellular level. I had great relief from the aloe alone, similar to the relief I felt from the metabolic juice enzymes. Taken together, they became a pretty strong anti-inflammation treatment. (Go to *www.TheTickSlayer.com/ aloe,* to learn more about this aloe.)

HBOT
(Hyperbaric Oxygen Therapy)

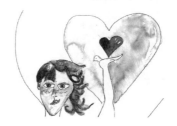

*"The most important thing in illness
is never to lose heart."*
– Nikolai Lenin

D r. Kalesh had a Hyperbaric Oxygen Therapy (HBOT) chamber. I decided to give it a whirl as the surgery was making me feel flat. HBOT deliverers oxygen to a person in a pressurized chamber and I knew I needed the oxygen to combat the oxidative stress in my body. The HBOT process increases the oxygen concentration up to 20 times more than normal at the cellular level, which promotes healing.

I controlled my claustrophobia and went into this capsule, but about 5 minutes into the depressurizing, my ears were hurting badly, and I just didn't feel good. So, I aborted the mission. It's purported to be effective for some people with degenerative type diseases, but I was going to do something a little more radical.

Blood Ozone

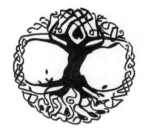

*"Every tomorrow has two handles. We can take hold of it
by the handle of anxiety, or by the handle of faith."*
– Author Unknown

Blood ozone therapy uses ozone ($O3$) to kill pathogens circulating in the blood and to boost your body's defenses. Ozone can be combined with intravenous chelation therapy which is used to treat arterial disease and heavy metal toxicity. Any type of oxygen therapy can be used to make tissues in the body more resilient.

The first few times I had the treatment, I felt like I was in a science fiction movie. A large syringe is filled with O3, which is injected intravenously. It's a little freaky because you're pumping air into your vein which can be dangerous if done fast, so the administration of the 50cc of ozone that was pumped in took about 50 minutes. After the blood ozone treatment I would get pretty sleepy and a little loopy, but after a good nap I would awake refreshed.

During this time, Dr. Kalesh attended a seminar to learn a new way of administering the blood ozone therapy. For my third treatment, I volunteered to be the guinea pig for his intern trying this new technique for the first time. This intern, an ND with a high aptitude, was totally cute so I couldn't say no! As I lay on the table, a needle went into my arm and the blood was drawn into a glass container on the ground using gravity. Then the same container was filled with O3, and the blood and ozone were mixed by gently shaking. The container was raised to allow the blood to flood back into my arm. This method seemed much easier on the body, so instead of getting sleepy at first, I got energized instead.

Though ozone therapy can create more free radicals when neutralizing pathogens I believe it, in conjunction with antioxidants (either orally or by IV), can be extremely helpful for treating any illness. The trick to preventing free radical damage is to make sure the treatments are given only a couple days (1-2 days) a week so that the body can normalize itself.

Blood ozone treatment sounds scary, but the German Medical Society for Ozone Therapy gave over 5 million treatments in the 1980's for people who were terribly ill with cancer and similar diseases. Only 40 cases reported side effects and there were only 4 deaths, making it one of the safest medical therapies of all time, especially when thousands of Americans die every year from drug interactions and reactions. Among people 35 to 54 years old, unintentional poisoning caused more deaths than motor vehicle crashes[1]. The actual

1. Centers for Disease Control and Prevention, National Center for Injury Prevention and Control. Web-based Injury Statistics Query and Reporting System (WISQARS) [online]. (2010) [cited 2010 Nov 30], Available from URL: www.cdc.gov/injury/wisqars.

number is hard to pin down as poisonings from prescription drugs and other substances are classified in medical records as injurious or accidental deaths. Millions of people in the United States have in-hospital adverse drug reactions (ADR) to prescribed medicine[2]. Dr. Richard Besser, a 13-year veteran of the Centers for Disease Control and Prevention, has stated that tens of millions of unnecessary antibiotics are prescribed annually for viral infections[3]. The estimated number of deaths caused by conventional medicine is an astounding 784,000 per year[4]. When people think of "German," they often think of Volkswagens, David Bowie and Wiener Schnitzel (well at least I do), but hopefully people will start recognizing them as pioneers in medical advances as well, like ozone therapy.

Ozone therapies are allowed only in certain states, so find out if your state allows them. Talk to your elected officials, and demand availability because no one should have to drive to another state to get something they should be able to get in their own neighborhood.

(To find out more about ozone home treatment, please see **Appendix XXVI**.)

2. Lazarou J, Pomeranz B, Corey P. "Incidence of adverse drug reactions in hospitalized patients". JAMA. 1998; 279:1200-1205.
3. Eliza Bussey. "CDC Warns About Overuse of Antibiotics," Reuters Health. May 9th. and Timothy Naimi, Pascal Ringwald, Richard Besser, Sharon Thompson. "Antimicrobial Resistance". http://www.ncbi.nlm.nih.gov/pmc/articles/PMC2631843/pdf/11485665.pdf (accessed February 14th, 2012).
4. US National Center for Health Statistics. National Vital Statistics Report, vol. 51, no. 5, March 14, 2003.

Blood UV Therapy

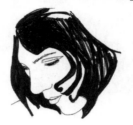

*"Turn your face to the sun
and the shadows fall behind you."*
– Maori Proverb

Also around this time, I tried Ultraviolet Blood Irradiation, a procedure where blood is removed and passed through a tube containing a UV light and then returned into your arm. The theory is that the UV light (which uses the full power of the energy spectrum), stimulates the fighter cells in the blood and in the process the immune system is strengthened (as are various enzymes), while pathogens are killed. Just a little blood that's been irradiated affects all the blood it comes in contact with. Some of the benefits of using this therapy include: improved circulation and oxygenation of tissues, anti-inflammatory effects, stimulation of the immune system, increased tolerance of the body for chemotherapy and radiation treatments, cardiovascular protection and increased anti-infection properties.

Blood Ozone and Ultraviolet Blood Irradiation are two fantastic ways to strengthen your immune system and these treatments were done after my final surgery to strengthen my own defenses. They also provided the final blow to my ordeal with Lyme disease, in part because what I did was not only get rid of the Lyme but I also killed the other pathogens that needed to go. I believe that most of the human population is carrying at least one type of virus, bacteria, pathogen, fungus and/or mold. I just think it only becomes evident when people finally succumb to their health issues.

In the Homestretch

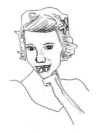

"For my part....I am a realist, but somehow,
optimism always keeps breaking out."
– Pierre Trudeau

The last phase with Dr. Kalesh was to test again for candida and take fluconazole (as a last resort) to get rid of it once and for all when the test results came back positive again. In addition, I used a progesterone cream to help me with my high estrogen level (and the inability to detox estrogen well), kept getting the nutritional IVs and did some of the other new therapies, such as Blood Ozone and Ultraviolet Blood Irradiation, which were most helpful. I also had a short chelation, via IV, to treat the heavy metals issue.

Is it Over?

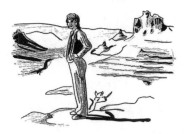

"We don't receive wisdom; we must discover it for ourselves after a journey that no one can take for us or spare us."
– Marcel Proust

Getting treatment was hard simply because I wondered when it was ever going to be really over. I didn't realize that a dental visit was going to take months to recover from. I was terribly ill for 7-10 days after the surgery and then I slowly came around with the use of the other treatments. For the following few months I worried that it would take years to recover. Not so, but it did keep me from training again. I simply could not go on. Although it really wasn't a choice at all; it was the second hardest decision I've ever had to make, right behind leaving West Point to pursue my athletic endeavors.

For days, I sat on my porch in the morning before the Florida sun got too intense to enjoy the day, watching the lizards run around on my screened in porch, in a daze. The Olympic Trials were in just a few months, and I had no more time to train. The 12 weeks I needed were gone. I had only 10, and I was still ill. I had told Coach Brooks I was tired of trying at this point. He told me that if I did quit track and field, that at least I had given it a good go. He was right, I had, but that just didn't sit right with me. I felt like I wasn't totally done, but had to accept my current fate.

I made the decision to take care of me first, and anyone who is ill will have to come to this conclusion: you can't take care of anything or anyone else if you're ill. You have to decide it's ME time and give yourself the time to heal. And that's what I did.

I sat on that porch and cried every morning for weeks until I returned to South Carolina to see my parents. I felt like a huge failure again. This blow may have been worse than at the 2005 US Track and Field Championships when I realized I was sick in the middle of my race. The good news is that I wrapped up my final treatments with Dr. Kalesh and went home to give my body the final full recovery time that it needed. Sure enough the last lingering symptoms started to disappear.

In retrospect, had I not gone down to Florida to try for the 2008 Olympics, I may not have discovered my last answers. Going down to Florida and trying to go for it again is what ultimately led me to a final complete recovery. It was the final push that got me over the top.

Miracle in a Box

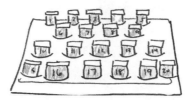

"Education is not received. It is achieved."
– Author Unknown

Iwanted to keep getting better although I knew my problems were pretty close to being over. I was in maintenance mode. Since I was on the path to a full recovery finally, I was interested in staying that way... forever. I was interested in finding out how I could keep the ideal levels of nutrients in my body on a continual basis.

I was still trying to recover from the surgery, and I still felt weak. I wanted to recover fast so I kept going back to my blood test to see what was out of balance. It's important to know that if just one nutrient, for example, is not balanced in the body, a person can get sick. Everyone who gets ill is deficient in essential nutrients.

After doing some research on my own, I found out a

person's body chemistry changes daily, depending on external factors like stress or internal factors like diet. Continually unbalanced nutrients add stress to the body as it works hard to correct the imbalance. The frustrating part of getting blood work to find the imbalances is that the test is expensive, and body chemistry changes daily, so the values might not always be correct by the time you get results (often weeks later). Honestly, I found this annoying and I needed to find a better way. I happened on a book by Lendon Smith, *Feed Your Body Right*[1]. This doctor treated all kinds of kids with ADD by simply correcting their body chemistry. In his book, Dr. Smith praised John Kitkoski, a chemist who developed an at-home program to balance body chemistry by creating smell sensitive vitamins, taste sensitive minerals and taste sensitive electrolytes. The kit contained all of the nutrients considered essential to the human body.

My grandfather, the retired physician, used to give people injections of certain vitamins when they were deficient. This was way back when doctors used the basic principles of health to heal people and did not just write them a prescription! I can't tell you how many ear doctors I went to growing up with earaches due to wax that just needed to be cleaned out and/or my undiagnosed food allergy, but instead of having these issues treated I was sent home with a prescription or was told I was a hypochondriac.

So I called up the late Kitkoski's surviving sister and said sign me up for the health program. Within a week I had my electrolytes, vitamins and minerals, and I jumped right in.

As an athlete I always thought that I knew what

1. Smith, Dr. Lendon, Feed Your Body Right. Understanding Your Individual Body Chemistry For Proper Nutrition Without Guesswork, New York: M Evans & Co, 1994.

electrolytes were. I always thought I was getting them by salting my food or drinking sports drinks. Electrolytes are made up of 7 key ingredients all of which all have a part in keeping the body balanced and "charged." Electrolytes keep the heart ticking and other vital components working properly. They keep infection out and also help the body detox waste on the cellular level. Just like many people, I had two huge misconceptions about electrolytes. I thought I could get them from sports drinks, fizzy packets, tablets, etc. While you can get some of these same ingredients in those products, you can't balance your electrolytes by taking these products. Sports drinks and gels replace glucose, which is important for maintaining energy levels, but they contain sugar which cancels the electrical potential of electrolytes. Electrolytes are positive ions of potassium, sodium, calcium, magnesium, and negative ions of chloride, bicarbonate and phosphate.

One of my concerns is that I've always had a low heart rate and low blood pressure and I felt fatigued just lying or walking around. I never got boosts of energy unless I was running or workout out, but within two days of balancing my electrolytes, this problem, once diagnosed by a former doctor as incurable, went away and I've never had it since I started taking a weekly maintenance of electrolytes. I've also heard of people with high blood pressure having outstanding results after they balanced their electrolytes. Elevated levels of sodium create electrolyte imbalances which have been linked to high blood pressure and heart problems. The impact of low sodium receives almost no attention. Low levels of sodium can lead to low blood pressure and create susceptibility to bacteria such as staph and E. coli. I believe that balancing electrolytes with a medical grade solution has far reaching effects on our health beyond the obvious issues I've mentioned here. Electrolytes give the body the electrical charge that keeps the heart, muscles and nervous system working properly. So, on a fundamental level they are the essence of life and become life giving to people who have electrolyte imbalances.

I also started taking the minerals in the kit. Minerals are elements found in all tissues and body fluids. They are involved in all body processes like proper bone development, nerve maintenance, hormone production, insulin regulation, liver function and fatty acids and cholesterol synthesis. Vitamins are just as important as they maintain and repair all body systems. Two essential nutrients in the vitamin kit that I had never previously given much thought to were: betaine HCL and ammonium chloride. Many people are missing the hydrochloric acid in their stomach that is needed to break down food properly. I used my sense of smell (as the vitamins were formulated so that each individual could use their olfactory senses to judge their need) to find the vitamins I was deficient in. Testing myself for HCL has been extremely beneficial as I go through temporary periods of needing it, just like most people do. Ammonium chloride plays an important role in maintaining the acid-base balance (human homeostasis better known as pH, which is vital to health). It has a stabilizing effect on nitrogen retention, which increases muscle protein synthesis. (Obviously great for athletes and non-athletes alike!) I found that the more people have been physically active in the past, the greater the need for supplementing with ammonium chloride. But, it's important that it's taken ONLY when needed, so being able to smell it and know when to take it has many benefits.

To find out more about Kitkoski's program, see **Appendix XXX**.

If I could go back in time, these products would have been my first step in treating my Lyme disease. I would go far enough back to start taking the kit as a child. Looking back, I have been deficient in one thing or another my entire life, which isn't uncommon but can lead to health conditions later in life. Even a body as deficient as mine was (even while taking all kinds of miscellaneous supplements my entire life), will still respond quickly when it gets the right tools to rebuild itself. It just goes back to the fact that our bodies really want to be healthy and the drive our body has to balance itself and to acquire the right building blocks is nothing short of amazing.

Back in South Carolina

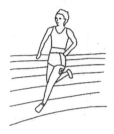

"There is no telling how many miles you will have
to run while chasing a dream."
– Author Unknown

B ack in South Carolina, I felt defeated. I had been so close to my dream, and once more I had to let it go. At this time I wondered if I was ever going to run again. I was just tired of trying and had no more "mojo." My coach was disappointed, my friends were disappointed, my family was disappointed, but I was crushed. I felt like a total loser-- I was a failure, again.

I kept taking the kit and I decided even though I felt good enough to jog, I just didn't have the desire anymore. I had nothing to work towards. The 2008 Olympics were coming in a few weeks; my teammates and friends would be there, and I was at home when I should be eating chow fen wearing the Red, White and Blue. I thought the Olympics would never end. They seemed to keep going on forever. Every time I went to a restaurant or to get the oil changed in my car, they would be on TV, just following me. I didn't read the paper during this time, nor did I watch TV. I tried to shut the world out so that I wouldn't even know the Games were going on. To this day, I still don't know how anyone fared. I was so crushed, but the good news is that the feeling didn't last. Eventually, I picked up where I left off. It wasn't until early in 2009 that I regained my spirit and was able to see what an amazing turnaround I had actually performed.

Yes, it's the End of the Summer!

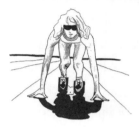

"Patience is the ability to count down before you blast off."
– Author Unknown

While everyone was wishing it would stay, I was glad summer was moving on. The Olympics were over, and I felt a sense of relief although I was still sad. My friend from high school was celebrating her 30th birthday by riding her bike from Pittsburgh to Washington, DC. Her new husband, an astute comic book fan with a very good sense of humor, was going with her. I was invited to go along and was glad to look forward to something physically challenging. I hadn't been on a bike in ages and to make it more difficult, I didn't get on one until we started riding. We rode the Allegany Trail and the C & O Canal, a mountain bike path (part of it was formerly an old railroad) that stretches across the country.

The first day was hell. I thought I would never make it, thinking that maybe I had not fully recovered yet from my health issues. We rode 60 miles that day and rode into a small Pennsylvania Amish town. By 7 p.m. when we arrived everything was closed, even the restaurants. (Finding food was a chore during the entire trip, and I had to feast on convenience store food for the first three days). The next morning I could barely move. Everything hurt, and my ass was sore, but the second day turned out to be easier than the first, and by the last day, I was feeling great. We laughed and rode along for miles on end. My body acclimated fast to the biking and the trip was a blast. I realized it was time to start training again. I began working out and trying to regain my overall fitness again by running and biking most days out of the week. I knew it would take a little while to build my fitness base again as I had lost every bit of fitness that I had spent years trying to build up. I was at the bottom, but I was just happy to be able to go for it again.

Gearing Back Up

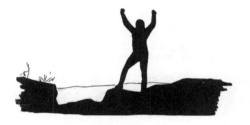

"What would you attempt to do if
you knew you could not fail?"
– Dr. Robert Schuller

In November I was easing back into things and decided to test myself. I trained intensely for 5 days back-to-back. Each day, I went to my max until I hit exhaustion. It was at that time that I knew the worst of my illness was history because being able to recover fast is a sign of good health.

By February my time trial in the 1600m was one of the fastest efforts in the United States for that early in the season. I ran a 4:38 in sub-optimal weather (with temperature in the 40's). I was thrilled and so happy most days that I couldn't finish a workout without crying, overjoyed that I had my body back better than it had ever been before. I started to do strenuous workouts that I was never quite physically mature enough to handle before.

Six months after the surgery in Texas my body was still expelling the infection left in my mouth. Each morning I had a little bit of drainage that I would spit out, but each month it became less and less, and by March 2009 it was completely gone. It took one full year just as Dr. Glaros said it would.

What I've learned is that if you don't keep moving forward, you will inevitably fall backwards. Would have, could have, should have; those are the words that scare me most. I don't want to go through life saying them. I've always wanted to live without regrets. I cannot say that I regret being bitten by the tick. For all I know, I was bitten as a child and grew up with Lyme disease. I'm just sorry that I didn't know about the disease when I found the tick on me in 2003, which wasn't treated until two years later. Had I been informed about tick diseases, I would have sought help immediately.

Lyme disease became an opportunity for me, something that is probably hard for most people with Lyme disease to actually hear. Hundreds of thousands of people are living life, many in excruciating pain, doing exactly what their doctors tell them to do and never getting better. There is no room for complacency when it comes to our own health. I believe if someone with Lyme disease can make it out of that accompanying psychotic mental state without harming themselves or others and have the desire, belief and will to attack it with all methods available until it's gone, it's certainly doable.

Having Lyme disease made me take a good look at my own health and what I wanted to do to change it. It made me desire all of the simple things in life even more. It renewed my quest in my sport of track and field, and challenged my spirit.

I got lucky that it hit me at a time when I was mature enough and smart enough to find my own answers…coincidence? I don't think so. From my experience I'm healthier than I've ever been in my entire life and I'm armed with the knowledge to keep it that way. You simply cannot be terrified of the unknown and you can't be afraid to succeed either.

This chapter in my life is officially closed. This Tick Slayer can finally retire and I'm back to the track, where I belong, competing to see how far I can go in this body, in this lifetime.

Epilogue:
Are You Ready for the Cure?

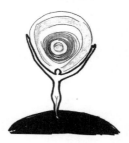

"What we think determines what we feel,
determines what we do, determines who we are."
– Author Unknown

Someone who is sick is going to run into several problems. First, you have to deal with the reason you became sick in the first place and your personal and emotional problems because I don't believe most people who get sick don't have some type of major stress. Everyone is different; one tiny stress for someone might be a HUGE stressor for someone else.

You have to get over the past before you can heal fully from disease. It's so much easier said than done for those who have a burning desire for revenge against someone who has wronged them or is just upset at life's ups and downs. Dr. Bob, the eccentric doctor from the Blue Ridge Mountains, told me that he wouldn't see people who didn't really want to be healthy. This perplexed me at first because I thought anyone who was sick wanted to be healthy at all costs, but it's actually not true. He told me that I wouldn't believe how many people went there to get help when everything else had failed but deep down inside they weren't truly ready to heal.

Some of the questions I had to answer before seeing Dr. Bob were about my goals and my reasons for getting healthy. Wouldn't you find it interesting if your doctor asked you this? Now I realize all doctors should ask their patients these types of questions and perhaps offer the emotional support and/or proper programs to address this issue. I think for many people it's just easier to stay sick.

Yes, it took me a lot of work to get over Lyme disease. I'm not saying it's easy, but I do say it's 100% doable. But how far are most people willing to go? Yes, I had to spend some money, but in retrospect most of the people I know who have Lyme disease have spent WAY more than me (and most are still very ill)! Perhaps it is the fear of failure that keeps people stuck on their merry-go-rounds. It's so easy to make excuses when you're not fully committed to something, but when every part of your mind is singularly focused on finding the answer, you'd be surprised at how fast answers can come. Looking back I'm surprised at how certain people came into my life at certain times.

When you're facing fear of the unknown, the best remedy is to simply take action. When it comes down to the nitty-gritty, most people have no idea what they are truly capable of.

Appendix I

IMPORTANT: The information included in this book is for informational purposes only. It is not intended nor implied to be a substitute for professional medical advice. The reader should always consult his or her healthcare provider to determine the appropriateness of the information for their own situation or if they have any questions regarding a medical condition or treatment plan.

Any opinions or recommendations expressed by third parties are solely those of these parties and are not the opinions, recommendations or necessarily the views of the author or publisher. Additionally, some third parties have compensated the author or publisher in exchange for inclusion in this book and the opportunity to present their opinions and recommendations.

Appendix I
Western Blot Lyme Test Results

There are multiple criteria supporting a positive test for Lyme disease. A test deemed positive has certain antibodies to B. burgdorferi and is very conservative, requiring 5 to 10 bands, or antibodies, for a positive result. Bands 23-25 kDa, 31 kDa, 34 kDa, 39kDa, 41 kDa, and 83-93 kDa are the indicating bands (kDa indicates the molecular weight). IgM, which tests a recurrence of persistent infection, can be a more sensitive indicator of exposure to B. burgdorferi, because of the risk of re-exposure and recurrent disease, this test can remain positive for a long time.

My IgM was positive for 30 kDa, 31 kDa, 39 kDa, 41 kDa, and 58 and 66 kDa, all of which are non-diagnostic. The overall IgM result with its conservative readings gave me an IND (indeterminate) for Lyme. My IgG, most notably bands 23 kDa and 41 kDa, which are the real tell-tale for a true indication (considered highly reactive bands), came back positive. I did not have enough positive bands overall for my IgG to indicate an active infection so it too was labeled IND.

Many Lyme doctors will agree that while an overall Lyme test may return negative or indeterminate results, when it comes to bands, a hit is still a hit, no matter how many bands show positive.

Appendix II
Neurological Issues Associated With Lyme disease

Neuroborreliosis is when a person's nervous system is infected with a spirochete (a cork screw looking type of bacteria) of the genus Borrelia. The bacteria cause an infection, in which inflammation also occurs. With Lyme disease, there are multiple strains of bacteria (called co-infections) that can be present alongside Lyme disease, simply because ticks (a main carrier of Lyme disease) often carry multiple types of bacteria.

Some of the symptoms of this infection include: facial paralysis or Bell's palsy, meningitis, shooting pains, memory loss, severe headaches, skin sensitivity, light and sound sensitivity, just to cover a few. Some symptoms are consistent with that of amyotrophic lateral sclerosis (ALS, also referred to as Lou Gehrig's disease). ALS is a form of motor neuron disease where the motor neurons that control voluntary muscle movement degrade.

Appendix IIIa
Standard Blood Test with Dr. Rachel

The most notable results from my blood test were: My basophils were on the low end, although still in the reference range. Basophils are a type of rare white blood cell. They contain material that the immune system needs when your body is under attack from infection or inflammation.

In addition to having a weak positive on my lupus panel, my C4 serum was 16 on a scale of 16 to 47. My C3 serum was also at the bottom of the scale. C3 and C4 are proteins in blood serum and their measurement gives you an idea of how well your body's defense mechanisms are doing to protect you from infections. Very low C3 or no C3 has been linked to fungal and parasitic infections. Increased levels, on the other hand, are linked to inflammation and inflammatory disease. My test results confirmed that I had an infection or rather, infections, many of them.

Abnormalities of C3 and C4 can mean: multisystem rheumatic disease, glomerulonephritis, hemolytic anemia or recurrent or overwhelming infection.

Decreased levels are associated with autoimmune disease.

My carnitine ester was WAY below normal. (Carnitine transports fatty acids across the mitochondrial membrane and is important in maintaining mitochondrial homeostasis.) Mitochondria are known as powerhouse cells because they provide cellular respiration, meaning "energy."

My B12 was also very low, and my carbon dioxide was way below normal. Carbon dioxide is important in the body and low levels can make you severely fatigued (just as having low B12 makes you feel fatigued). All this meant my cells were having a very hard time producing energy!

I was also borderline iodine deficient (putting all the pieces together later, I realized that I have a bit of thyroid issue as well). This is yet another thing that will make you EXTREMELY tired. To really drive home the point that I was severely "deflated," I also had really low glutathione, which is needed for beating infection because it's a super antioxidant and protects the liver from toxins. If your body is ravished of it, you'll feel like crap. Later, I would find out that I could have started correcting this by getting injections of glutathione and taking supplements like milk thistle and N-acetyl cysteine (NAC) which act like the raw materials that your body needs to produce its own glutathione naturally.

Appendix IIIb
Standard Blood Test with Dr. Kalesh

Standard blood tests usually include: a lipid panel (which is helpful in ruling out problems with cholesterol and fat issues), a complete blood count (CBC) and a metabolic panel.

My results indicated that I had an infection in my gut (which I already knew). Dr. Kalesh went over this pretty quickly, looking for anything out of the ordinary. After seeing the test results he recommended getting a vitamin B complex, but the IV already included this, so I was covered. My mean corpuscular volume (MCV), which is the measure of the average red blood cell volume, was high suggesting hemolytic anemia. Alcoholics often have a high MCV, but so do people who have a vitamin B12/folic acid deficiency. Some doctors will use the MCV to guess if a patient has anemia, and though low levels may suggest anemia, a ferritin test measuring the actual storage of iron will help make that determination.

The test results were not to my liking. I knew some values were skewed because of infection, but I kept studying my values and later on come up with my own conclusions.

My blood urea nitrogen (BUN) was low, although it was in the reference range, perhaps an indication of low nitrogen. The BUN test measures the amount of nitrogen in your blood resulting from the waste product urea. Urea is made in the liver and is passed out of the body in urine. The BUN test shows how well your kidneys are working. If the kidneys aren't working well, the BUN level rises. Liver damage or disease can lower your BUN level, but a low level could also indicate low protein in the diet, poor absorption, a wasting disease, or a liver impairment. Since I already had a good understanding of the waste problems that come from detoxing issues, it made sense that my liver might be overburdened.

My calcium was also low but within range, as was my total protein, but my globulin was low and out of range, suggesting immune deficiency, malnutrition, liver disease, anemia or poor protein digestion. And my A/G ratio, the proportion of albumin to globulin, was really high, perhaps indicating fibrinogen. Because I didn't keep in touch with Dr. Bob, I never knew how to keep on the soy enzymes I was taking previously for this.

Another concern was my AST (SGOT), which was high but within range, perhaps indicating a liver problem, or an issue with infection or Epstein-Barr virus (mono). Aspartate aminotransferase (AST), one of the liver enzymes also known as serum glutamic oxaloacetic transaminase (SGOT), is a protein made by the liver cells; when these cells are damaged, AST leaks into the blood. So a high AST level usually means there is some liver damage.

Appendix IV
Thyroid Function and Indications of Thyroid Dysfunction

The thyroid, a butterfly shaped organ in your neck, directly effects your metabolism. If your metabolism isn't working well, the result is poor health. The thyroid energizes cells in the body by stimulating mitochondria. Low thyroid indicators are: brittle hair and nails, dry skin, fatigue, sleep apnea, susceptibility to ongoing infections, weakness, slow heart rate, joint pain and high blood pressure, to name a few. The low energy output gives people the feeling of being cold all the time.

It's important to consider getting your triiodothyronine (T3), thyroxine (T4) and thyroid stimulating hormone (TSH) tested. Low levels of T3 and T4 are indications that you do no have enough thyroid hormones.

Appendix V
Bio-Identical Hormones and Adrenal Exhaustion.

There are a lot of reasons why people's hormones go whacky. Illness is one. Hormonal systems like the adrenals and thyroid become exhausted because of toxin overloads occurring in the kidneys, liver and lymphatic system. These organs are needed for toxin elimination and need these precious hormones.

Getting your hormones balanced by way of bio-identical hormones (BHRT) is one solution to replace what your body is having a hard time manufacturing due to illness or age. Bio-identical hormones are not the same as synthetic hormones, which are thought to cause diseases like cancer. These hormones instead are compounded and made specifically for each individual in a form that is found in nature so that your body not only responds to it, but can utilize it correctly.

Having a cortisol imbalance is very taxing on the body. Cortisol (a very important hormone) is made in the adrenals and high levels mean your adrenals are maxed out, giving you the feeling of moods you cannot control like anxiety, fatigue and depression. Cortisol helps our energy levels, digestion, joint fluidity, inflammation control, boosts the immune system and much more.

My levels of cortisol were low, making me feel depressed and flat-out exhausted. High levels can indicate an adrenal crash in the process, as adrenals will produce more cortisol to counter stress. Baldness (or too much hair), being underweight, cravings for salt and sugar, allergies, difficulty getting aroused for sex, lack of concentration, and low blood pressure are some indications of high levels of cortisol.

Some other hormones to have tested and corrected are: estrogen, testosterone, progesterone, pregnenolone, DHEA, Human Growth Hormone (HGH), thyroid, and insulin in addition to cortisol.

Appendix VI
Testing Liver Enzymes for Detoxing Capabilities

The DetoxiGenomic™ Profile by Genova Diagnostics® is a blood test that evaluates a person's ability to detox environmental toxins and identifies adverse drug reactions. Environmental toxins include; pesticides, herbicides, pollutants, solvents, heavy metals, pharmaceuticals and nutraceuticals, and also waste products produced by the body. The test can also identify a person's predisposition (stemming from impaired metabolism) to disorders such as: ADHA, alcoholism and psychiatric disorders such as bipolar disorder. It can also identify risks for diseases such as different types of cancers and neurodegenerative disorders like Parkinson's and Alzheimer's.

I had several polymorphisms (mutations) detected in two genes crucial to Phase 1. Decreased Phase 1 clearance causes toxic accumulation in the body. Adverse reactions to drugs are often due to decreased capacity to detox. (That might explain my psycho behavior under Dr. James' massive antibiotic therapy.) For these genes I was flagged on car exhaust, cigarette smoke, charbroiled foods, and learned that the burning of any type of organic material will make me "weak in the knees" as my body will have a very difficult time trying to detox.

The suggestions for helping me minimize risk were to get lots of aerobic exercise and cold water fish, for example. I was to stay away from car exhaust and industrial solvents and not eat any well-done meats. And of course not smoke!

Other suggestions to help me increase Phase 1, but also to help Phase 2, were to eat cruciferous vegetables (cauliflower, broccoli, Brussels sprouts, watercress and cabbage) and to eat more vegetables and fruits (soy, grapes, onions, black tea, green tea, herbs), and certain spices (basil, turmeric, cumin, poppy seeds and black pepper). Improving Phase 1 and Phase 2 detoxification explains why eating more vegetables and fruits protects against cancer. With Lyme, think about how unbelievably toxic we get from traditional antibiotic therapy and then the die-off on top of that! It makes sense that we would need to improve our detox capabilities.

Helping Phase 2 meant my body would be able to better "dump" the toxins through urine and feces. When I got this test done, I realized that my body was screaming to detox due to the vomiting of bile. That was a big mystery for me, this vomiting of a putrid yellow mess, and now I knew why and what exactly it was.

This is where it gets even more interesting. There are several different processes that work in Phase 2. The first one, methylation, breaks down neurotransmitters, dopamine, epinephrine (I had a scare with this one at my dentist later on), and norepinephrine. I found out I have a hard time breaking down estrogen; I may also be at risk for neuropsychiatric disorders and late-onset alcoholism. I've always had bad PMS and wondered why but getting some answers like this made be feel good. I could understand how my own specific body chemistry worked.

The suggestions were for me to avoid alcohol and minimize mental and environmental stress. These types of stress directly affect the break-down of my estrogen. It was also suggested that I ensure an adequate intake of B vitamins, magnesium and protein.

The next Phase 2 tested was acetylation. This process detoxes environmental toxins, like smoke and exhaust. The enzymes responsible for this process were genetically impaired (again, due to genetics and evolution, we all have some type of impairment. But, knowing what we have and doing something about it can keep us healthy). I was to increase intake of vegetables and fruits to help this along.

The third Phase 2 process tested was gluta~~ conjugation. This isn't the same as just having y~~ glutathione levels tested. This process shows how well your body can detox solvents, herbicides, fungicides, lipid peroxides and heavy metals by way of glutathione conjugation. Anytime any of these genes are impaired, it means more of a toxin burden and increased oxidative stress for that individual.

I had a null reading for one gene in this process. I needed to take glutathione supplements to raise my glutathione levels naturally. The other suggestion was eating the fruits and vegetables mentioned earlier. I was also to avoid insect sprays, industrial solvents, fungicides, and herbicides. I remember at West Point being handed a bottle of DEET and I just couldn't get myself to put it on. My gut feeling toward it was bad. When in doubt, always use your gut instinct if you can.

Last, oxidative protection was tested. I had a double chromosome variation for one gene. This varied gene affected mitochondria, which didn't make me too happy because this is where energy is basically produced. The enzymes responsible for protecting my cells against free radical damage were slightly dysfunctional.

The suggestions for helping my body cope were to take antioxidant supplements to raise glutathione levels, such as vitamin C, N-acetyl-cysteine, alpha-lipoic acid and milk thistle. I gravitated towards these supplements naturally as well as to the suggested kinds of fruits and vegetables. I love berries and anything that has a high antioxidant value (like yerba mate, green tea, black tea).

in C that I began had a dramatic effect

test might explain why it helped me so

lly helped me dump my waste build up

Appendix VII
IV Vitamin C

Vitamin C in high doses can be extremely helpful in treating people with infectious diseases. Even if vitamin C does not cure a specific infection, it can resolve many conditions to some degree. Dr. Albert Szent-Gyorgyi, the scientist who won the Nobel Prize in 1937 for his discovery of vitamin C, asserted that energy exchange can only occur when there is an imbalance of electrons. Vitamin C acts as an ongoing electron donor, keeping the electron flow at an optimal level; therefore, making it useful as a treatment for anything infected, like dead tissue, that can no longer maintain the flow of electrons (that healthy tissue does)[1].

IV vitamin C (often referred to as "high" C, because of the dosage) is used to treat people as an alternative to Chemo, young children with autism, and those with autoimmune diseases.

Vitamin C is just one of the body's natural chelating agents that are responsible for such things as the digestion, assimilation, and transport of food nutrients, the formation of enzymes and hormones, and detoxification of toxic chemicals and metals.

---

1. Dr. Thomas Levy. "Curing the Incurable: Vitamin C, Infectious Diseases and Toxins" http://www.tomlevymd.com/books.html

Appendix VIII
"Tsi-Ahga" For Enhancing the Immune System

Tsi-Ahga is a form of 3-beta-D-glucans. It's a type of beta-glucan derived from conks that grow on certain cone-bearing trees. According to one naturopathic doctor, the 3-beta-D-glucans which make up part of the cellular structure of these conks cause an increase of T-cells, macrophages and neutrophil white blood cells when ingested. Studies have shown that the number and viability of these particular cells is increased by as much as "4000% within 20 hours after taking Tsi-Ahga[2]." I used a blend of black cumin, stabilized rice bran, muscadine grape, Tsi-Ahga and the heart of garlic. Each one is demonstrated in scientific research to strengthen, support and modulate the immune response in different ways. It stands without question that if the immune system is strengthened, numerous ailments and illnesses can be aided and alleviated.

You can order Tsi-Ahga at:

www.TheTickSlayer.com/TSI

Appendix IX
Acupuncture

Acupuncture is the practice of inserting small needles into the body's surface to influence the physiological function of the body. It's a practice that has been used in China for the last 5,000 years. Bodies have an energy grid that is electrical. Acupuncturists use needles in specific places to move energy along these pathways.

2. Philip Couldpiller Landis, NAP, N.D., "Real Answers to Real Question, Restoring the Sacred in Healing" pg. 96.

They believe when these pathways become obstructed, deficient, excessive or unbalanced it causes illness.

Moxibustion is a complimentary treatment in which Moxa (also called mugwort herb) is burned on top of some of the needles to create a heating effect and stimulate circulation of energies.

Appendix X
Thermal Imaging

The physician report for my images said: Head and Neck: Myofascial hyperthermia is noted bifrontally and at the neck bilaterally. There are no thermal findings to indicate sinus, temporomandibular joint (TMJ), dental, thyroid or carotid artery dysfunction (but Dr. Bob disagreed with this finding about the dental part).

It went on to say: There is no thermal evidence to suggest carditis related to Lyme disease. (At this point, this might not have been the main issue and my gut said something bigger was the main problem. I'm sure at this point I still had Lyme floating around, but the human body can carry all types of strange viruses, bacteria, organisms and still regulate itself normally.)

Back: Myofascial inflammation is noted on upper back. Hyperthermia outlines the lower thoracic and lumbar spine, suggesting diffuse joint disease.

Abdomen: Increased thermal activity is noted on right and left upper quadrants and may relate to hepatic/ spleen dysfunction.

Lower Extremities: Loss of the expected patellar hypothermia is consistent with joint dysfunction involving knees. (I admit the image was inflamed around my knees, and may have been inflammation due to Lyme).

Appendix XI
Live Blood Analysis

Dr. Bob gave a score from 0 (best) to 10 (worst) based on what was visually represented.

I was given a 5 for thrombocyte aggregation and lymphocytes and chylomicrons. This wasn't very good as platelet aggregation can contribute to cardiovascular disease and is an indication of circulation problems, capillary blockages, blood clotting issues and other problems associated with the heart. I was given a 2 for plaque and oxidized cholesterol. I got an 8 for hypersegmentation of white blood cells (these cells maturation process is slower than normal and these cells are considered pathological) and hemolysis (Red blood cells that have broken open). Hemolysis can lead to conditions like anemia.

He also gave me a score of 8 on parasites. Parasites are not only prevalent, they can migrate from the colon to everywhere else in the body[3]. They can be found in your blood, muscles, skin and organs. One more interesting note is that Dr. Bob said I had an amoeba based on my blood analysis and that I probably got it out of the country (yep, I didn't think that the medication given by those Bolivians killed all of those nasty boogers).

I also got a score of 8 on metals. We get metals from

3. Centers for Disease Control and Prevention, Parasites- Blood, http://www.cdc.gov/parasites/blood.html (accessed November 7, 2011).

cookware, dental work, pipe solder, table salt, smog, contaminated fish and other common things. Metal buildup may be found in the fatty tissue, the brain and the nervous system. Degenerative diseases like Alzheimer's, MS and Parkinson's have been linked to heavy metal overload. I basically had mercury poisoning.

Other notable scores were a 5 for vitamin C assimilation and 5 for inflammation. I also got a 6 for circulatory system, which indicated that my system was either depleted or overburdened. It can be easily overburdened by waste build-up.

Luckily, I got 0s for eight other items.

Appendix XII
Metabolic Enzymes

Saccharides, found in fermented soy enzymes are necessary for optimal cellular communication and are effective in supporting the immune system. These molecules mediate most of the communication that occurs between the 100 trillion plus cells in the human body, which is important since defective cell messages may have implications for immunity. Some purported benefits by those using fermented soy enzymes are:

• Increases oxygen levels and neutralizes free radicals by raising PH levels to more alkaline levels.

• Helps you preserve your body's own antioxidants to be used elsewhere other than the digestive process.

• Provides energy directly to cells by enhancing your body's own electromagnetic fields.

• Helps protein molecules split, helping your body's

digestion- undigested matter gets eaten up.

- Promotes a healthy blood environment and improves the energy supply to cells.

To get these enzymes visit:

www.TheTickSlayer.com/enzymes

Appendix XIII
Blood Sugar Support

Receptor sites are areas on the cell that pick up and receive hormones and different nutrients and chemicals. Receptor sites may become clogged from coming in contact with chemicals and toxins. People today are exposed to so many toxic agents and chemicals that their receptor sites become choked, this is when the ability to assimilate nutrients becomes diminished and blood sugar levels can inch up. This can create pre diabetic conditions in people. People who are pre diabetic (or type 2 diabetic) cannot metabolize carbohydrates properly.

Either the body does not produce enough insulin or the cells ignore the insulin. Insulin is what takes the sugar (food) from the blood into the cells. When glucose builds up in the blood instead of going into cells it can lead to diabetic conditions.

The neuropathy that is associated with diabetes is due to high amounts of insulin in the body which causes inflammation. Research has shown insulin resistance is also a risk factor for other diseases, including hypertension and cardiovascular disease and now cancer[4].

---

4. Monika Guttman, "Resisting Insulin, The hormone insulin, a key part of diabetes, may be the real culprit in everything from cancer to Alzheimer's disease." http://www.usc.edu/hsc/info/pr/hmm/06fall/insulin.html (accessed November 8, 2011); Miranda Hitti, "Why Belly Fat Hurts the Heart," http://www.webmd.com/heart-disease/news/20080129/why-belly-fat-hurts-the-heart (accessed January 24th, 2012).

Improving the body's sensitivity to and ability to use insulin can keep blood glucose levels normal, therefore producing less insulin and ultimately slowing the body's inflammatory response.

To get the diabetes pack I used to clean my receptor sites, visit *www.TheTickSlayer.com/bloodsugar*

Appendix XIV
Rife and ONDAMED®

Many people with Lyme disease use Rife machines. There are many types of Rife machines (named after Royal Rife, an inventor who claimed he could render viruses that he believed caused cancer inert by using resonances or frequency). Rife machines use electro-medicine to kill harmful microbes.

In the electro-medicine field is the ONDAMED, whose website states, "works by using mild sound and accompanying magnetic pulses to stimulate the body at various frequencies. A medical practitioner monitors the response of the autonomic nervous system to these frequencies by noting changes in the pulse and informs the patient of findings, thus providing the information needed for biofeedback to occur. The identified stimulating sound and magnetic frequencies are then temporarily applied to specific areas while the patient relearns how to be in a healthier state. A key feature of ONDAMED is that relaxing frequencies are part of the re-education process. Many studies have shown that tension and stress reduce feelings of wellness and the addition of relaxing frequencies help re-establish the proper balance between the sympathetic nervous system and the parasympathetic nervous system." Visit *www. TheTickSlayer.com/ondamed* for more information.

Appendix XV
Parasite Cleansing

There are numerous parasites in everyone, but in unhealthy bodies they may prove to be a huge burden on the body's immune system and overall health. Some signs of having a parasite problem are: diarrhea, abdominal pain, fatigue, blood/worms in the stool, and itchy anus. Some other signs that may be less noticeable are: nausea, stomachache, irritability, skin conditions, anemia, joint pain, gas and bloating and weight issues (losing too much weight or having a ravenous appetite without weight gain).

A stool test, like a GI Panel can assess the probability of parasites in the digestive tract, but parasites are not bound to the digestive tract. They can be found in the skin, brain, muscles and other organs. Common misconceptions about having parasites are that those who travel or own pets are the ones who are susceptible, but everyone can get parasites just from normal living activities as they are found in the soil, food, water and even air. By eliminating parasites yearly, people can enhance their energy and overall health by decreasing their toxic load, boosting their immune system and absorbing food better.

Cleansing can be an important part of getting your health back, but when doing parasite cleanses, for example, the result of the removal of a high load of parasites, could make a chronically ill person's body produce more insulin, so glucose levels should be closely monitored in people who have diabetes.

To get the cleanse I use once a year, visit:
www.TheTickSlayer.com/parasitecleanse

Appendix XVI
Coffee Enemas

Coffee enemas can be done with an enema bag or with a disposable enema bottle from your local drug store. The disposable enemas usually come with a solution in the bottle. This should be discarded, you only want the bottle.

Caffeinated coffee without flavorings should be used. Brew the coffee by any method; however, I think the best results come from brewing the coffee on a stove top. You can bring the coffee and water to a boil, let it sit and then boil it again (double boiling is said to help extract more of the beneficial compounds in the coffee). A few tablespoons of coffee grounds in about 14 ounces of water should suffice.

Once the coffee has cooled and has been filtered from the grounds, it goes into the enema bottle or bag. After inserting it in the colon you should lie down on your back for 15 minutes and then you can remove the tube and go to the bathroom.

Appendix XV11
Probiotic Enemas

Probiotic enemas are a great way of introducing beneficial flora back into the intestines, bypassing the digestive system. Many cancer patients use these enemas to repair their guts after chemo. In my opinion, one of the quickest ways to fight candida (the overgrowth of yeast, a major health issue that comes from taking pharmaceuticals) and reestablish homeostasis in the gut is to do these probiotic enemas.

For more information on the probiotics I use, go to *www.TheTickSlayer.com/probiotics*

Appendix XV111
Colon Cleansing

A colon cleanse can refer to lots of different methods of cleansing the colon. It can be as simple as changing your diet for a specific length of time (lots of water, vegetables and fiber, or a juice only fast), or seeing a colon hydrotherapist where the entire length of your colon is irrigated gently to remove all waste. Coffee enemas act as a small colon cleanse as they only irrigate a small part of your colon.

I believe the best colon cleanses are the ones that are diet specific and include herbal formulas (in powder form) that help loosen and remove unwanted material from the colon (but can also have a huge cleansing effect on the liver). People who have distended bellies may want to get a series of colon irrigations done in addition to making dietary changes. It's important to make sure you see someone qualified to give these treatments as it can be dangerous.

If you have a chronic disease for which you are taking medication, make sure that your medication will not adversely affect you if your condition were to suddenly improve as a result of cleansing your body.

To find out more about the colon cleanse I do yearly, visit: *www.TheTickSlayer.com/cleanse*

Appendix XIX
Liver Flush

Orthophosphoric acid is an inorganic mineral that is commonly used for gallbladder and liver flushes. It has other uses as a concentrated acid with corrosive properties, but is safe to take internally when diluted. It has the ability to remove calcium and lipids (fats) from arteries and improve cholesterol metabolism. The drops I used for my liver flush contained orthophosphoric acid, inositol and choline bitartrate. The phosphoric acid when mixed with apple juice (which contains high levels of malic acid) can soften gallstones. Inositol and choline help prevent the accumulation of fats in the liver and are used in many liver aid formulas.

To get the formula and instructions on how to do a complete liver flush, visit *www.TheTickSlayer.com/livercleanse*

Appendix XX
Ayurvedic Medicine

Ayurvedic medicine (also known as Ayurveda) originated in India thousands of years ago. It's the practice of balancing one's body and spirit to prevent illness and promote wellness. Specialized diets, herbs and massage are used to cleanse and restore this balance.

Appendix XXI
NT Factor®

The formula in NT Factor contains phospholipids and glycolipids which help each cell absorb more nutrients to produce energy with via the mitochondria organelles.

To learn more about NT Factors, visit: *www.TheTickSlayer.com/NT*

Appendix XXII
Glutamine for a Healthy Gut

Glutamine is an amino acid that is an amide of glutamic acid (which means it gets converted to glutamic acid in the body). It plays a role in protein synthesis, is a cellular energy source and helps in the Krebs cycle (the body's way of producing energy). The gut loves glutamine, as do the kidneys, for balancing acid and immune cells.

Even though many athletes take glutamine during training to combat illness, injury and stress, it is also marketed to athletes for muscle growth but there is no evidence to support that use.

Appendix XXIII
GI Panel

A GI Panel is used to screen for bacteria, fungi, yeast and other parasites. In addition, it screens for enzyme levels and for food intolerances to common foods. Lastly, it can provide a measurement of how healthy the gut is by evaluating inflammation and immunity.

Appendix XXIV
Candida Cleansing

Candida can be a problem in anyone who has taken antibiotics, or just has a poor diet. Many people with Gluten intolerance have many of the same symptoms as people who have an overgrowth of candida. Limiting or completely eliminating processed foods like candy and breads is part of the plan to combat candida. Taking probiotics orally and via enema is a proven way to reduce the candida population. Lastly, supplements that are designed to reduce yeast populations can be a helpful addition. View my current picks at: *www.TheTickSlayer.com/candida*

Killing candida, just like killing other organisms like bacteria and parasites, can produce "die-off" in which the organism releases an endotoxin that the body has to dispose of. When candida die in large amounts, symptoms similar to bacteria die-off can occur; therefore, consider performing a detox regimen before and during this treatment.

Appendix XXV
Gut Health

There are many products that contain different nutrients to support intestinal mucosa. Mucosa is the barrier in the intestines that absorbs nutrients and prevents the passage of toxins. Breakdowns in this barrier can cause all types of conditions such as dysbiosis, nutrient deficiencies, Irritable Bowel Syndrome (IBS), etc. Amino acids, essential fatty acids and phospholipids (such as vitamin E, L-glutamine, N-acetylglucosamine (NAG), gamma oryzanol and phosphatidylcholine) are used to support this mucosa and improve overall gastrointestinal health. Some of these nutrients can be found in whole food sources. Gamma oryzanol is found in rice bran oil. Lecithin is a nutrient that is rich in phosphatidylcholine. Some foods that contain high amounts of phosphatidylcholine are wheat germ, egg yolks, fish and brewer's yeast.

You can find out more at:

www.TheTickSlayer.com/gut

Appendix XXVI
Ozone Therapy At Home

An at home ozone unit can be used for odor and pathogen elimination in the air and water and to clean air and water without any nitrogen by products. The pH of water stays neutral and the O3 has no adverse affect.

My unit contained a UV lamp and ozone generator and had the ability to hook up to a medical grade oxygen tank for more therapeutic uses. It also had an air diffuser stone that was an easy hook up to go from air to water. Some people use the diffuser stone to ozonate olive oil and use it for medicinal purposes. The general rules for my unit are to run the ozone an hour per every 1000 cu. ft. (10ft. L x 10ft. W x 10ft. H) or less of room space. For water, it's generally 15 minutes for each gallon.

To view the unit I have, go to
www.TheTickSlayer.com/ozone

Appendix XXVII
Removing Metals

There are two ways to test for metals. One is by hair analysis, which can be done at home. (See *www.TheTickSlayer.com* for a hair analysis home kit.) The other method is by testing a urine loading sample after a chelating agent has been administered via IV by a medical doctor. Chelating agents are substances which bond to metals, minerals and chemical toxins in the body, allowing offending substances to be disposed of via urination and defecation. Chelating agents, such as ethylenediaminetetraacetic acid (EDTA) are used to grab heavy metals and fatty plaques. EDTA is one of the most common agents; however it cannot chelate mercury, which DMSA and DMPS (two other chelating agents) do.

Appendix XXVIII
Joe's Gadgets

Infrared saunas create heat that is a narrow band of energy within the 5.6 to 15 micron (μ) level. This type of energy travels only 2-3" deep into the body to increase circulation and nourish damaged tissue. Infrared heat is used to stimulate tissues and organs, helping the user to gently perspire out toxins. It is also touted for its ability to increase blood circulation by widening blood vessels and strengthening the cardiovascular system. Since detoxing is a major component of increasing one's health, infrared heat is becoming increasingly popular. Many people with Lyme suggest it as a major treatment to reduce pain.

Joe's ozone steam sauna combined the power of ozone with that of steam. Steam surrounds the body and opens the pores of the skin so that the ozone can be introduced through the skin and into the bloodstream where it can travel to the lymph nodes and fat tissue. Cleansing the lymphatic system is very important when dealing with chronic illness. It is an effective hyperthermia treatment, which is the artificial inducement of fever to boost the immune system. Other benefits of note are the relaxing of muscles, oxidizing toxins and elimination of toxins, boosting blood circulation, pain relief, elimination of bacterial and viral infections and the speeding up of metabolic processes.

To view an array of infrared saunas and ozone saunas, like Joe's, visit *www.TheTickSlayer.com/sauna*

Appendix XXIX
Natto for Blood Health

Natto is made from fermented soybeans and is of Japanese origin. Natto reduces the likelihood of blood clotting as it contains an enzyme called Nattokinase, which may be helpful for people predisposed to heart attacks, strokes or thrombosis. It is thought to have mild fibrinolytic activity when taken orally, which means it can help dissolve fibrinogen (fibrin clots).

Appendix XXX
My Miracle Kit- Blood Chemistry Balancing

The Smell Sensitive essential vitamin, mineral and electrolyte kit contains everything that is considered an essential nutrient in the human body. These formulate the basic building blocks for other nutrients that are created by the body for optimum health.

35,000 people were included in a study by chemist John Kitkoski to determine the effectiveness of his product[5]. 'Smell Sensitive' means each person can determine which supplements they should take by smell alone. Those that smell good to mild indicate the body has a need for that vitamin or supplement. Those vitamins that smell bad indicate the body has an adequate or excess amount. The vitamin kit contains: Vitamin A 10,000 I.U. of A from fish liver oil, Vitamin B-1 100mg. of (Thiamine), Vitamin B-2 100mg of (Riboflavin) Vitamin B-6 100 mg of (Pyridoxine Hydrochloride), Vitamin B-12 500 mcg of (Cyanocobalamin), Vitamin C 250mg of (Ascorbic acid), Vitamin #7 Smell Sensitive Vitamin D 400I.U. of D from fish liver oil, Vitamin E 200I.U. of (d-alpha tocopherol), Vitamin H 300 micrograms of (d-Biotin), Choline 300mg of (Choline Bitartrate),

5. Elsie Kitkoski, Electrolyte LLC, "Spectrum for dietary supplementation selection system and method following human olfactory," fax, Feburary 7, 2012

Calcium 83.3mg of Calcium for 10grains of (Calcium Lactate Pentahydrate), Folic Acid 400 micrograms of (Folacin), Betaine HCL w/Pepsin (pepsin 1:300 N.F.-13mg), Inositol 300mg of (hexahydroxycyclohexane), Iron 27mg of (ferrous fumarate), Magnesium 133mg of elemental Magnesium from Magnesium Carbonate, Vitamin B-3 100mg of (Niacin), PABA 100mg of Para-Aminobenzoic Acid, Vitamin B-5 250mg of (Pantothenic Acid) from d-Pantothenate, and Ammonium Chloride 7½ grains of (sal ammoniac).

The electrolyte kit is formulated so that each person can determine their individual need for replacement and contains three different formulas for normal, low and high blood pressures. Once electrolyte balance is lost, drinking plain water won't help! Drinking plain water will dilute electrolytes or create greater electrolyte imbalances. Mineral water contains a variety of minerals that can further skew the balance of electrolytes. Sports drinks provide mostly carbohydrates, not electrolytes.

Their milliequivalent formula will provide electrolytes without upsetting the body's mineral balance or adding carbohydrate calories. It is an isotonic, medical grade electrolyte replacement with sodium, potassium, chloride, phosphorus, bicarbonate, magnesium and sulfur.

The mineral kit balances your ratio of minerals based on your unique body chemistry via taste. It contains the six essential minerals in taste sensitive formula: potassium phosphate, zinc sulfate, magnesium chloride, copper sulfate, potassium chromate, and manganese gluconate.

To get more information on this body chemistry balancing kit and how to order, visit *www.TheTickSlayer.com/kit*

Appendix II

IMPORTANT: The information included in this book is for informational purposes only. It is not intended nor implied to be a substitute for professional medical advice. The reader should always consult his or her healthcare provider to determine the appropriateness of the information for their own situation or if they have any questions regarding a medical condition or treatment plan.

Any opinions or recommendations expressed by third parties are solely those of these parties and are not the opinions, recommendations or necessarily the views of the author or publisher. Additionally, some third parties have compensated the author or publisher in exchange for inclusion in this book and the opportunity to present their opinions and recommendations.

Appendix 2-I
Biological Dentistry by William P. Glaros D.D.S

Current observations and studies by top health care providers reveal that two factors, toxicity and chronic infection, are often at the root of people's health conditions. The source of this toxicity and infection is often found in a place one is not inclined to look, the mouth.

Many medical professionals, including dentists, are unable to respond to questions like these:

• Are biotoxins from bacterial agents having a synergetic effect with your heavy metals, jaw lesions or dead teeth?

• Is the bacteria most associated with Lyme Disease (Borrelia Burgdorferi) causing your symptoms or is the severity of your symptoms related to your current individual immune response?

• Could removing mercury fillings, nickel-based crowns, dead teeth or chronically infected bone possibly affect your disease?

......Yet patients shouldn't give up so easily.

For Perry Fields, the life-changing reality of her disease compelled her to ask the tough questions and explore the potential roots of her condition.

The people that do the best are well prepared for their biological dental visit. They are nutritionally fit for their type and condition. They are usually working with an MD, ND, DC, or other health care provider who is knowledgeable about natural health issues and the potential roles that dental disturbances can have on health.

Most biological dentists are comfortable with the concepts of energy meridians running through the body, connecting oral sites to the rest of the body. Principles of acupuncture would teach that a disturbance on an energy meridian of the body could cause dis-ease along that meridian. A disturbance could be electrical, magnetic, bacterial, viral, or fungal. We clearly are applying our post-doctorate training to deal with dental aspects of these issues.

The oral surgery procedures of cleaning out infected extraction sites or other lesions in the bone is often requested. The proceeds of these sites varies with the conditions that caused them. It is our practice to send the specimen from the surgery sites to the Pathology Department of the University of Texas Dental School for a biopsy. The incidence of cancer at these sites is extremely rare, and we are expecting more to find out if the site is a marrow defect, osteonecrosis, osteoporosis, or the like.

If you have the drive to pursue this direction, utilize Perry's experience: Study the issues at hand. Review your medical and dental health history parallel to your symptoms. If you are inclined to address the dental issues, look for a biological dentist and interview that office for similar protocols and treatment patterns that experienced practitioners follow.

God bless you on your journey. Let's cheer Perry on as she runs her race.

As much information as you want on these subjects can be found using Perry's resources, our web site listed below, and by internet search.

For more information on biological dentistry go to: *www.BiologicalDentist.com* or contact Dr. Glaros' office at: (281)-440-1190

Appendix 2-II

ONDAMED: A non-disease label approach to improving body functions versus treating disease by Rolf Binder, Inventor & Silvia Binder, N.D., Ph.D.

An approach that rapidly allows you to find the hidden physiological and emotional cause of your symptoms while simultaneously stimulating your nervous system with specific therapeutic fields. Some of the benefits include:

- Enhancing metabolism in cells & cellular environment
- Affecting different kinds of tissue including soft tissue, cartilage, and even bone
- Improving lymphatic flow
- Strengthening immune functions
- Affecting the autonomic and central nervous systems by infiltrating impulses in the brain wave patterns.

How it works: The human body works on the basis of bio-physics and bio-chemistry. While traditional medicine has much to offer in the chemical sense, it lacks the therapeutic approach of physics. Practitioners use the non-invasive ONDAMED technology and the biofeedback loop to scan the body for underlying dysfunctions, such as inflammation, infections, scar tissue and emotional trauma residing at a cellular level. These areas often prove to be the source of disease and symptoms that might be otherwise difficult to find. Identified areas are treated with specific pulsed electro-magnetic fields to stimulate tissue and the nervous system. Stimulus with ONDAMED specific pulsed fields helps reduce local stress and improve metabolism and lymphatic flow resulting in reduced inflammation, pain and swelling, while improving stress tolerance by reducing cortisol levels and by influencing the nervous system.

Within minutes, the ONDAMED therapist finds the specific treatment stimuli for the patient, finds the actual location that is in need to receive the therapy and treats the discovered area by applying a systemic therapeutic stimulus. The stimulus energizes the flow of electrons across natural immune system inflammation barriers. These barriers are often undetectable or untreatable in any other way, and include free radical scavengers.

When placing the non-intrusive applicator to a specific area, electrons and white blood cells are summoned to the area to start the repair process. ONDAMED, therefore, jump-starts the body's immune functions and directs the immune response to the area of dysfunction, which is often hidden or in "stealth mode" to the immune system.

Tissue vibration can enable detoxification of unwanted heavy metals, waste and toxins, potentially resulting in improved metabolic functions. Nutrients, remedies and supplements can then be assimilated by "cleaner" or detoxified tissue and cells.

The lymphatic system (an important part of the immune system) can also be stimulated. Toxins and waste can then be discharged by stool, urine, sweat and the release of fluid in other areas such as the eyes by discharging tears.

The ONDAMED epigenetic impact is now being

considered, and while we appreciate that no energy system or even medications, can bring about a cure of any disease, ONDAMED shows that the body can be stimulated to heal itself.

Fortunately, the ONDAMED practitioner may often discover the influence of "out of balance" diseased cells and tissue when they pick up the response signaling of the autonomic nervous system from the patient's issues. We therefore, enjoy great expectations for the future of ONDAMED.

ONDAMED encompasses the individual's specific needs at the time of discovery by finding the patient-specific treatment stimulus, the exact location that needs stimulation and non-intrusively delivers the stimulus during the same session, often providing immediate results.

ONDAMED is very unique in its ability to deliver specific resonant frequencies to the source of illness. ONDAMED approach is focused on what we discover about the illness and its location, and is both practitioner and patient friendly.

To read more of this article and to discover more about Dr. Binder's successful use of Ondamed on her son's thrombus, go to: *www.TheTickSlayer.com/ondamed*

For practitioner information or to find an Ondamed practitioner near you, visit *www.Ondamed.net* or call +1-845-534-0456

Appendix 2-III
Intravenous Vitamin C by Thomas E. Levy, MD, JD
Overview

The administration of vitamin C by vein is an enormously potent weapon in the arsenal of the open-minded clinician. Infectious diseases, poisonings or toxin exposures, and nearly all chronic degenerative diseases will reliably show dramatic positive responses to sufficiently dosed vitamin C. Most acute viral infections can be completely cured in short order by enough intravenous vitamin C over a period of several days. Non-viral infections also respond very well, as vitamin C can directly attack the microbe, augment the effects of traditional antibiotics, and stimulate the immune system by multiple mechanisms.

Because of the pro-oxidant nature of all poisonings and toxin exposures, vitamin C also serves as the ideal antidote for any and all acute intoxications. Different toxins respond to different degrees to vitamin C therapy, but vitamin C will, first and foremost, save any victim of poisoning, since the damage is always done by an overwhelming onslaught of free radical production and increased oxidative stress. It just has to be given soon enough, often enough, and in adequately high doses.

Intravenous vitamin C is also proving to be an exceptional anti-cancer therapy. It is probably the ideal chemotherapy agent for the entire gamut of cancers. Regular chemotherapy drugs poison all cells, accounting for the many and severe side effects seen with so many cancer treatment protocols. Vitamin C, however, targets the cancer cells specifically while invigorating and nurturing the surrounding normal cells. Cancer cells, with their elevated hydrogen peroxide and free iron levels, are literally sitting ducks waiting for vitamin C to catalyze the production of hydroxyl radical via the Fenton reaction, killing the cell in very short order. Normal cells, however, do not have the intracellular microenvironment of the cancer cell, and they thrive on the administered vitamin C while the cancer cells die. Vitamin C also augments the effects of regular chemotherapy, as long as the dosing of the vitamin C is not absolutely simultaneous with the chemotherapy, as the chemotherapy is typically also a highly pro-oxidant toxin, or poison. As long as the chemotherapy can enter the target tissues before the vitamin C enters the blood, it can do its damage to the cancer, while the vitamin C can prevent or lessen the side effects inflicted on the normal cells.

An Intravenous Vitamin C Protocol

Generally, vitamin C should probably be administered in sterile water or normal saline. There is no good reason to give it with glucose (for example, 5% dextrose in water), as this just adds something to the blood to directly compete with the vitamin C for entry into the cell. The more glucose is available to the cell when the vitamin C is given, the less vitamin C will enter the cell. This occurs because the glucose and vitamin C molecules are very similar in structure. In those animals that make their own vitamin C, glucose is the substrate molecule that is converted to vitamin C. Because of this, high doses of vitamin C, mistaken by the body as a large amount of glucose, can sometimes stimulate a large release of insulin from the pancreas when rapidly infused, causing symptoms of hypoglycemia. This is rarely of consequence clinically, and it is usually enough to let those patients eat during their infusions rather than to infuse glucose with the vitamin C at the outset of the infusion in "anticipation" of a possible insulin surge.

The optimal amount of vitamin C to be infused depends on a number of factors. Important factors include patient age and body size, along with the diagnosis and how acutely and critically ill the patient is when first seen. Very acute infections and critical cases of poisoning should be treated aggressively with high doses of vitamin C, generally given relatively rapidly. Individuals with more chronic conditions can be given lower doses, infused more slowly.

For acute infections and acute poisonings, a very general dosage guide would be a starting dose of about one gram per kilogram of body weight, given over sixty to ninety minutes. This would be from 20 to 25 grams for a 50-pound child and 100 grams for a 220-pound adult. Depending upon clinical response after the first infusion, subsequent infusions could be scaled up or down in dosage. Infections and poisonings impairing consciousness may need several hundred grams of vitamin C in the first 24 hours to assure a positive clinical response.

50 to 150 grams of vitamin C can be mixed with 500 cc of sterile water. The highest concentration that

vitamin C can have in water is 500 mg/ml. In extremely critical situations, where death appears imminent, this concentration can be administered by syringe as a direct IV push, potentially giving 5 to 15 grams of vitamin C over a one- to five-minute period. The IV push can provoke a substantial hypoglycemia, which could require the administration of glucose by vein if significant enough.

When a patient with cancer or other chronic degenerative disease is being treated, doses should be initially low and slow, until individual sensitivities have been determined. A G6PD deficiency, which can result in a hemolytic anemia when vitamin C is first administered, can be readily checked by blood test. If such a deficiency is present, taking several grams of liposome-encapsulated glutathione by mouth for an hour or two before the IV should stabilize the red blood cells enough to tolerate the vitamin C infusion.

If G6PD status is normal, the cancer/chronic disease patient should still receive the first infusions over three to four hours. If these are well-tolerated, then subsequent infusions can go much more rapidly, allowing the blood concentration of the vitamin C to peak at higher levels, increasing target tissue levels.

Adjunctive Measures

Regardless of the condition being treated, it's always a good idea to use as many ways of delivering vitamin C to the body as possible. Several grams of liposome-encapsulated vitamin C orally, as well as bowel tolerance amounts of sodium ascorbate powder dissolved in water or juice, should be taken on a daily basis during the acute treatment period. Vigorous hydration is also important, although the patient usually develops enough thirst to keep this from being unduly neglected. Antibiotics and other medications can be given as prescribed during the vitamin C protocol.

A list of doctors, many of whom will give intravenous vitamin C, can be found at *www.acam.org*. Liposome-encapsulated products can be found at *www.thetickslayer.com/livon*. My books and more of my writings can be found at www.tomlevymd.com. A good source of sodium ascorbate powder can be found at *www.vitamincfoundation.org*. Thomas E. Levy, MD, JD, July 6, 2011, televymd@yahoo.com

About the Author

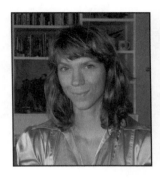

Perry Louis Fields grew up in South Carolina and began running at a very early age. She attended the Governor's School for the Fine Arts in high school in the visual arts. Her track and field endeavors led her through three colleges (including West Point). She graduated Clemson University with a degree in Packaging Science. She is an extreme outdoors enthusiast and a hobbyist golfer, poker player and rock hound. She has a thirst for knowledge in the areas of health and space. In her spare time she enjoys cooking, reading, painting and sculpting. Perry continues to serve as a coach to people who are suffering from chronic autoimmune illnesses. Perry can be reached at *www.TheTickSlayer.com*

Connect with the author:

Like this Book: *www.facebook.com/tickslayerbook*
www.twitter.com/perryfields

Acknowledgments

Thank you Dad. If it weren't for you, I wouldn't have experienced the joys of being an athlete. I'll never forget my first runs on those dirt country roads and the elation of winning my first fun runs.

Thank you Mom, for being my caregiver, supporter, and #1 ally through thick and thin.

Thank you Culla for your loving support.

Thank you Madaddy, for being a fine example of what a medical doctor should be and being a great grandfather to me!

Thank you to my grade school teachers and college professors who, as my mother says, DID know what to do with me. Your encouragement was invaluable.

Thank you to all the individuals & characters I met in the healthcare arena who helped me put parts of this puzzle together. Special thanks to all the maverick doctors and healthcare professionals I have yet to meet. Continue pioneering.

Get Health Recovery Coaching!

Do you or a loved one have an infectious or autoimmune disease? Did you read this book and are now wondering how to implement the information you've gained? Perhaps you just need an extra push in the right direction.

Consider getting health recovering coaching by Perry or one of her trained coaches so you can get to point A to Z as quickly as possible!

What to expect:

1. Referrals to favorite healthcare professionals
2. Mentoring to help you out of the "sticky" phases of recovery, where your improvement seems to plateau
3. Continuous Q & A access to your coach
4. Help with planning your recovery- how to merge the best "kitchen solutions" with traditional medical help.

Email: *info@theticslayer.com*

The Tick Slayer Order Form

Yes, I want to order _____ copy(s) of The Tick Slayer.
The Tick Slayer $24.95
Enclose $5 for shipping for one book (plus $2 for each additional book) ($10 outside the U.S.) and mail, or fax your name, address, zip, telephone, email and credit card including expiration to:

Postal Orders:

Zippy Publishing, LLC.

110 Liberty Drive, Suite 200

Clemson, SC 29631   Fax: 864-406-2013

Name _____

Address _____

City _____

State /Province_____Postal Code _____

Country _____Phone/fax _____

E-mail _____

_____ Cash, check, money order

Please charge my ☐ Visa ☐ M/C ☐ Amex ☐ Discover

Card # _____ Exp Date _____

For cardholders:

I authorize Zippy Publishing, LLC. to charge my card for the amount of: _____

Signature _____ Date _____

This book is available at quantity discounts for bulk purchases. For more information visit: *www.TheTickSlayer.com/bulk*

Fast and secure online ordering at: *www.TheTickSlayer.com*

Special, Speedy Recovery Plan for Those with Challenging Health Issues

I've condensed my knowledge and wisdom from my 5 year journey to a full recovery, into an 11 page plan that I would follow if I had to do it all over again. It includes my step by step recovery plan, my very best resources and guidance to help anyone who is struggling with a serious illness.

I took a lot of great steps, but not necessarily in the correct order. This is exactly what I wish I had when I first fell ill. It would have saved me a lot of agony, money and time. Enjoy! Wishing you a healthy, speedy, and full recovery!
- Perry Fields

You can purchase this comprehensive and all-inclusive plan and download it instantly. The value of this plan exceeds an hour long private coaching session with Perry ($350.00 dollars). Don't miss out!

You can order your plan by going to:
www.TheTickSlayer.com/plan

Share with Friends!

Please feel fee to pass along this book
to friends and family.

Sign up for Perry's FREE newsletter.
The Tick Slayer newsletter is a bi-monthly newsletter
focusing on Perry's health secrets, including real-life
examples of how she stays healthy and disease-free.
www.TheTickSlayer.com

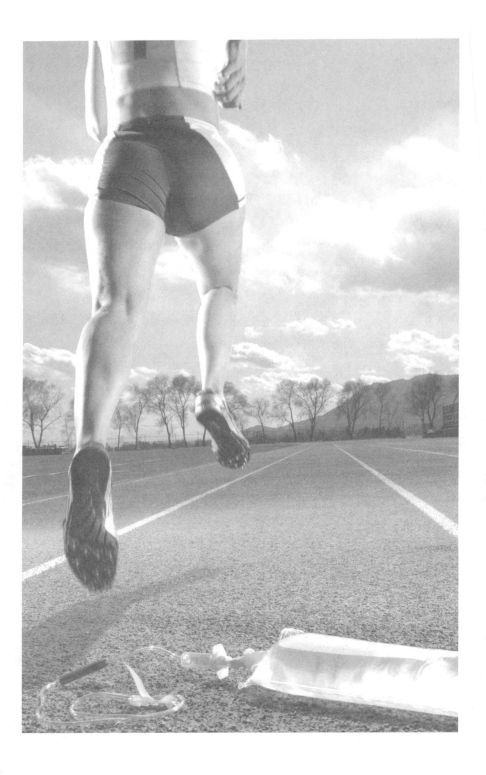